ACQUIRED TASTES

acquired

WHY
FAMILIES EAT THE WAY
THEY DO

tastes

BRENDA L. BEAGAN | GWEN E. CHAPMAN

Josée Johnston, Deborah McPhail, Elaine M. Power,
and Helen Vallianatos

UBCPress · Vancouver · Toronto

23 22 21 20 19 18 17 16 15   5 4 3 2 1

Printed in Canada on FSC-certified ancient-forest-free paper
(100% post-consumer recycled) that is processed chlorine- and acid-free.

LIBRARY AND ARCHIVES CANADA CATALOGUING IN PUBLICATION

Beagan, Brenda L., author
Acquired tastes : why families eat the way they do /
Brenda L. Beagan, Gwen E. Chapman, Josée Johnston, Deborah McPhail,
Elaine M. Power, and Helen Vallianatos.

Includes bibliographical references and index.
Issued in print and electronic formats.
ISBN 978-0-7748-2857-4 (bound). – ISBN 978-0-7748-2858-1 (pbk.). –
ISBN 978-0-7748-2859-8 (pdf). – ISBN 978-0-7748-2860-4 (epub)

1. Food habits – Social aspects – Canada. I. Chapman, Gwen E., 1959-, author
II. Johnston, Josée, 1972-, author III. McPhail, Deborah, 1977-, author
IV. Power, Elaine M., 1961-, author V. Vallianatos, Helen, author VI. Title.

GT2853.C3B42 2015   394.1'20971   C2014-905556-0
                                                 C2014-905557-9

Canadä

UBC Press gratefully acknowledges the financial support for our publishing
program of the Government of Canada (through the Canada Book Fund),
the Canada Council for the Arts, and the British Columbia Arts Council.

This book has been published with the help of a grant from the Canadian
Federation for the Humanities and Social Sciences, through the
Awards to Scholarly Publications Program, using funds provided
by the Social Sciences and Humanities Research Council of Canada.

UBC Press
The University of British Columbia
2029 West Mall
Vancouver, BC V6T 1Z2
www.ubcpress.ca

contents

PREFACE

THIS BOOK IS THE PRODUCT of a deeply collaborative effort spanning several years, from 2007 to 2013. Brenda Beagan and Gwen Chapman originally conceptualized the project and brought Josée Johnston, Elaine Power, and Helen Vallianatos onto the research team. Together, we refined the funding proposal over several months, a process that resulted in a successful submission to the Canadian Institutes for Health Research. Josée took responsibility for recruiting participant families and collecting data in Toronto, Elaine in Kingston and Prince Edward County, Helen in Edmonton and Athabasca County, Gwen in Vancouver and the District of Kent, and Brenda in Halifax and Kings County. In each site, research assistants did much of the recruitment, data collection, and preliminary analysis. Several skilled transcribers in the five sites worked with us to turn the recorded interviews into text. At UBC, Gwen worked with research assistants to maintain a website that allowed us to share all of our data.

Two years into the project, when Deborah McPhail joined us as a postdoctoral scholar, we had already begun coding and analyzing data. She became an integral part of the team, continuing to work with us well beyond the completion of her postdoctoral position.

As our analyses progressed, we all presented at various conferences and prepared journal articles from the study data. We also met routinely – in person and virtually – to discuss our findings and learn from one another. We were constantly challenged, pushed, and enriched by the ideas, theories, and bodies of research we encountered through other team members. At a team meeting in Toronto, we decided that the study needed a book format to showcase the complexity and interconnections in the stories of people who had talked with us. We generated the outline of that book together. Each of us worked on different chapters in various ways.

The Introduction was drafted by Brenda and significantly rewritten by Gwen. Chapter 1 was drafted by Gwen, with contributions by Brenda and Deborah. Chapter 2 was written by Josée with doctoral students Alexandra Rodney and Michelle Szabo. Similarly, Chapter 3 was written by Josée with doctoral student Sarah Cappeliez. Chapter 4 came out of a paper that Alexandra Rodney wrote for a course with Josée, and later they transformed it into the chapter, with subsequent feedback from Gwen and Brenda. Chapter 5 was written by Deborah, and Chapter 6 was drafted by Brenda and significantly improved by Elaine. Chapter 7 was written by Brenda with very substantial feedback from Gwen. Chapter 8 was written by Helen, with support from Brenda for preparing the data. Chapter 9 was written by Helen, with feedback from Gwen, and was significantly rewritten by Brenda. The Conclusion was written by Gwen and Brenda, using feedback from everyone.

Throughout the process, everyone read and provided feedback on the chapters. When the book started to come together, Brenda pulled it into something coherent, uniting the arguments, reducing the length of chapters, tidying the formatting, and integrating the references. She also made revisions during the peer review process, with feedback from Gwen.

We hope we have produced a text that readers will find as compelling as we found the stories of our participants!

ACKNOWLEDGMENTS

WE OFFER OUR HEARTFELT thanks to the 105 families across Canada that gave of their time and expertise in repeat interviews with us, which form the basis of this book. We hope we have done their stories justice.

We thank the research assistants who worked with us in various capacities during the years involved in this study and the writing of this book: Jennifer Black, Kate Cairns, Kaaren Christ, Jessica Diener, Brent Hammer, Melanie Kurrein, Kerry Mellett, Alexandra Rodney, Dean Simmons, Jamie Szabo, and Michelle Szabo. Postdoctoral fellows Sonya Sharma and Nancy Salmon both contributed in key ways at key moments in the project's unfolding, which we greatly appreciated.

We would like to thank the Canadian Institutes for Health Research for grant funding (operating grant 84425) that made this study and this book possible.

ACQUIRED TASTES

introduction

HOW DID YOU decide what to eat today? How did others in your household decide? How is your daily approach to eating determined by your budget? How is it affected by what foods are locally available, in stores and restaurants? More deeply, how is the way you eat influenced by what is seen as normal in your community? Among your friends and peers? How do you think your eating patterns may be affected by (largely unspoken) expectations about social class?

If various ways of eating are understood as normal for people from certain class backgrounds, how do you suppose you might use class-based expectations about food to display your identity as a member of a particular class? Similarly, if certain ways of eating are understood as normal for men and women, boys and girls, how might you use your everyday food practices to convey messages about your gender identity? Given that healthy eating is preached at you from virtually every magazine at supermarket checkouts, how do you engage with those messages? How is your engagement (or non-engagement) influenced by who you are – in terms of gender, geography, class, race, ethnicity, and age?

These questions lie at the heart of this book. We spoke with adults and teenagers from 105 families to discover how they talked about food, how they defined themselves through it, and what shaped their cravings, food aversions, and health aspirations. In the chapters that follow, we explore differing ways of thinking about food and why we eat what we do. But first, meet 2 of the 105 families on whose stories the book is based!

FAMILY FOOD PRACTICES: TWO CASE STUDIES

The Valverde Family

Bernice and Basil Valverde live with their seventeen-year-old son, Bart, in a renovated character home on the East Side of Vancouver, British Columbia.* Bernice (forty-three) holds a graduate degree and is an urban planner. Basil (forty-five) is a high-school teacher. They are a comfortable upper-middle-class family with an annual income of about $120,000.

Food is an important part of their life. They make a point of eating meals together at least three or four times a week, and Bernice describes cooking and eating as "so central to what it means to be a family ... We've built time into our schedules to make food. It's important to us." All three Valverdes are good cooks. Basil is perhaps the most skilled – he cooks dinner most week nights and specializes in Indian food. But Bernice enjoys reading recipe books, grocery shopping, and cooking on weekends, and Bart says he's "pretty good at" certain dishes such as tuna melts made in a waffle iron. He proudly states that he can cook a "mean steak." They share their interest in food and cooking with neighbours, who often join them for meals: "Cooking is a big part of our social scene ... It's a big part of how we gather socially."

The Valverdes are adventurous eaters who enjoy experiencing food from a variety of cuisines and who prioritize quality. Bernice notes that "we spend more money on food than most people ... We just decided that it's worth it." Concerned about the environmental impact of the industrialized food system, she prefers to buy local foods. She is also careful about what she and her family put in their bodies, buying mostly organic foods and avoiding highly processed ones: "I don't like

. . . .

* As will be explained later in this chapter, we employed pseudonyms for all study participants, selecting their initials to indicate their location. Here, the initials BV indicate British Columbia, Vancouver.

the chemicals. I don't like ingredients that I don't know where they come from ... Why wouldn't you choose something fresh and organic over something that is full of chemicals and colours and additives?" Bernice and Basil do periodic detoxifying cleanses to "cycle stuff out of your body, get rid of things ... It's really important that your body is balanced and things are cleaned out and given rests."

Even though Bernice describes Bart as "an incredibly healthy eater" who "will eat a wide variety of foods," she also acknowledges that as a teenager, he has been going through a period of dietary independence, eating white bread instead of brown, enjoying "low-brow" processed foods such as Miracle Whip, and convincing his parents to move back to eating meat after years of vegetarianism (Bart reports this latter change as one his father happily embraces!). Bart himself is unconcerned about healthy eating as he eats "a lot of fast food" and chooses to prioritize taste.

The Austin Family

Amy (forty) and Anthony (forty-two) Austin live with their children, Archie (fourteen) and Angelina (thirteen), in a small community in northern Alberta, about 150 kilometres north of Edmonton. Both parents have university educations; Anthony is a teacher and Amy works in an office. The annual family income is approximately $100,000. The Austins own a well-maintained ten-year-old split-level home near the edge of town.

For this family, food represents comfort, stability, and tradition. To the extent that their busy schedules allow, they try to eat evening meals with everyone together several times a week "because we need to still be a family sometimes" (Archie). Amy often prepares the meals, which she describes as "stay[ing] with the fundamentals" and her children describe as including "potatoes and a meat and then vegetables." In the past few years, since Amy took a job with longer hours, Anthony has more frequently prepared meals. Although he can be a more creative cook than Amy, he is "a little bit more relaxed" than she in his weekday preparation, using more prepared foods and serving "simple suppers like fish and chips and burgers." Overall, family members feel that what they eat is "normal food" and "not over the top." They often share meals with Amy's parents, who live nearby, but they rarely entertain friends. When Amy does cook a special meal for company, the menu is quite traditional for a rural Alberta family with a Ukrainian heritage, typically including turkey, perogies, "lazy *holubtsi*" (cabbage and rice casserole), two vegetables, Caesar salad, and a dessert.

When grocery shopping, Amy and Anthony prioritize low-cost food that meets their quality standards and preferences. Amy says, "I rarely, if ever, buy anything that's not on sale. Like rarely, rarely, unless it's an absolute essential that we need, like milk." At the same time, she also "look[s] for quality and how it's going to affect the body as well, yet we're not really stringent about it either." She repeats this relaxed approach to healthy eating in noting that family meals are "pretty balanced" but adds that "we don't count how many fruits and vegetables the kids have during the day or anything."

For Amy and Anthony, concerns about environmental and ethical issues do not enter into daily food decisions, although they acknowledge that living in a small farming community does shape how they think about food. They do some of their grocery shopping in local stores to support local businesses, and they always use canola oil because Amy's father is a canola farmer. However, they do not deliberately look for "local" or organic foods, and for much of the year, they eat produce from the garden that Amy maintains at her parents' home: "I freeze my vegetables for the winter. When I run out, I have to buy, but I'm not into the organic thing at all. I am into the fresh fruits and vegetables from the farm, though. I would *much* rather have something that I grew than what someone else grew, because I know what went into it."

Overall, for Amy, home-cooked meals are essential: "I would not feel like I was giving my family what they should have, and I would feel like I'm raising them to be unhealthy if I wasn't preparing their food for them." Anthony acknowledges that "it's not as important to me," but he and the two children also appreciate the family's traditional, relaxed approach to food.

WHAT SHAPES HOW FAMILIES EAT?

The Valverdes and Austins are real families who participated in the study presented in this book, although their names have been changed. Their approaches to food and eating display an interesting mix of similarities and differences. On the surface, the families seem quite alike, as both are headed by a heterosexual white couple in their forties, with similar educational backgrounds, professions, and incomes. But though both families value eating meals together and consider food to be important for health and enjoyment, their overall approaches differ markedly. The Valverdes are happy to spend money on an eclectic mix, emphasizing local, organic, and plant-based foods as much as possible. The Austins, who are much more frugal, do not mind using processed food and stick to a fairly traditional "meat and potatoes" diet. When they do eat local organic produce, it is because they or other family members have grown it in their gardens, not because of political or health concerns.

How did these similarities and differences develop? The Valverdes and Austins live in comparable economic contexts, where the costs of living and median household incomes are similar. They have access to equivalent education and media, and both represent the dominant Canadian cultural group. However, their geographic settings do differ – the Valverdes live in a metropolitan, multicultural, coastal city, and the Austins reside in a small, relatively homogeneous Prairie town. To what extent does this difference shape what they eat and how they talk about food? In what ways have other individual, social, or environmental factors been equally or more influential?

This book explores such questions. It examines the everyday food practices of families from a variety of social and geographic contexts, examining how they talk about what they eat and the beliefs, values, and concerns that shape their food practices. It uses a sociological lens to address the question "Why do we eat what we eat?"

These questions are of interest to a variety of audiences. Much of the interest relates to health, as scientific and popular literature clearly links diet with illnesses such as cancer and cardiovascular disease, in Canada and globally. Increasing rates of overweight and obesity, frequently accompanied by claims regarding the health risks of fat, have fuelled concerns about the need to improve the healthfulness of diets. There is growing evidence that understandings of the negative long-term health implications of obesity are at least as much social construction and moral panic as medical reality (for more on critical obesity studies, see Flegal et al. 2007; McPhail 2009; Biltekoff 2013). Nonetheless, with government, industry, and public support, extensive nutrition education has been provided through schools, social marketing campaigns, and the media, and policies have been developed to effect changes in food availability and access to nutrition informa-tion. Most Canadians report that nutrition is a "very important" con-sideration when they choose food, and up to a third see themselves as "very knowledgeable" about the subject (Canadian Council of Food and Nutrition 2009). Despite such overwhelming interest in health and diet, surveys show that few Canadians meet current nut-rition recommendations (Garriguet 2006). Clearly, a more nuanced understanding of food choice processes is needed to address diet-related health problems.

Understanding how people make their food choices is also of in-terest to a growing "food movement" that promotes environmentally sustainable, healthy, and socially just food systems (Food Secure Can-ada 2014). These concerns arise from the realization that what people eat affects not only their own health, but also the health of the planet – for example, greenhouse gas emissions are produced through food production, processing, and transportation; soil and water are con-taminated by industrial farming practices; and sensitive ecosystems are destroyed to provide land for intensive farming. As well, the eco-nomic well-being of rural communities and the physical, social, and economic well-being of food producers around the world are affected by the choices that people make when they buy (or refuse to buy) cer-tain foods. Players in the food industry are equally interested in what people eat. Farmers, food processors, the grocery industry, restaurant chains, and the supporting infrastructure depend on people buying the food that they provide.

And, of course, fundamentally, food matters to everyone. Almost all of us eat every day. We spend money on food. We devote time to buying, preparing, and eating it. It can give us pleasure, it can help keep us healthy, and it can make us sick. It can be a source of stress and anxiety if we don't have enough money and if we worry about its effects on our bodies or our ability to provide the "right" food for the people close to us. Within families, it can be a source of tension when family members have different goals and expectations relating to food.

The authors of this book share an interest in understanding how and why people make their food choices. As academics with expertise in sociology, anthropology, gender studies, health studies, and nutri-tion, we all believe that food choice is not just an individual process, a matter of personal taste. Individuals make decisions in the context of their social situation, their family and community, their cultural environment, and their local food milieu. Clearly, material realities such as availability of diverse, affordable, and high-quality foods and the economic means to purchase them are key determinants of what people eat. Yet other social and cultural processes are also at play. Foods carry differing meanings and associations for people in different social contexts, influenced by gender, race and ethnicity, age, class background, income, and education. These meanings are often place-specific, learned through locally available social discourses that constitute some foods as "good" or "bad," "healthy" or "unhealthy," "appropriate" or "inappropriate" for members of specific social groups. Food may be about physical sustenance, but it also has profound symbolic resonance, signifying one's class status, masculinity or femininity, family cohesion, caring, community, independence from parental authority, and resistance to cultural assimilation. Thus, individuals from differing social groups and specific places may employ distinct "cultural logics" when they are deciding what to eat.

Despite this theoretical understanding, however, insufficient empirical research has explicated the cultural logics at play in food decision making in specific places. We thus embarked on the research presented in this book – a study of how local food cultures, socio-economic status, and the family context interact to produce everyday food practices in urban and rural Canada. Our decision to explore these questions in families with adolescent children allowed us to examine how food meanings and habits are formed, transmitted, resisted, and transformed through multiple levels of social relationships – that is, not only through relations embedded in specific regions and communities, but also through the intense relationships *within families* between children and parents and among adults. Our focus on family food socialization is especially significant given what sociologists know about the role of parents in socializing their children to consume and appreciate certain kinds of culture and to reject other kinds as inappropriate, including food.

EATING PRACTICES AND SOCIO-CULTURAL CONTEXT: CONCEPTUAL TOOLS

Usually, people think and talk about eating practices as being individual choices or habits. Certainly, food practices are influenced by personal preferences, nutrition knowledge, practical concerns about time and convenience, and hunger and food intolerances, among other things. These factors are all important. Food activists and health promotion advocates are quick to point out that financial and material resources also affect what people eat: if they can't afford something, they are unlikely to eat it. Are there nearby grocery stores? Do they offer affordable, high-quality products? Can they be accessed by people who do not have cars? Do they carry items from a range of ethnic cuisines? Do they sell locally produced foods, organic foods? Is there a farmers' market nearby? What kinds of restaurants are close? Do people have access to land where they can grow some of their own food? In these and many other ways, material resources shape food practices.

The focus on individual, economic, and environmental influences, however, often overshadows attention to more social and cultural aspects that shape how people eat. It is clear that people are not guided solely by individual tastes, preferences, and rationales about food, or by how these interact with financial and material resources. Research shows that food habits of groups differ in patterned ways, including by age, gender, cultural background, and education (O'Doherty Jensen and Holm 1999; Johnston, Taylor, and Hampl 2000; Raine 2005; Garriguet 2006; Prättälä et al. 2007). As well, food habits differ for rural and urban people, and in varying parts of the country (Garriguet 2006; Shields and Tjepkema 2006). Although some of these latter dissimilarities may reflect differences in food environments, in our market-based globalized food systems, differences in food availability often reflect differences in local consumer demand.

In addition, what people *say* they know and believe about eating is not always what they *do,* even when a variety of foods are readily available to them (Caplan 1997). The measurable individual traits that are thought to predict consumption often fail to do so. And it is not always easy, or even possible, for people to explain their choices. The gap between what they say about food and what they actually do every day, their difficulty in articulating their decisions, and the patterns of eating habits of people in different social locations (the intersections of age, gender, race, ethnicity, class, education, income, and migration status) suggest that eating practices are affected by multiple, not-always-conscious, socio-cultural factors. We focus on these conscious, semi-conscious, and unconscious socio-cultural rules in this book.

In recent decades, social scholars have explored – both theoretically and empirically – the ways in which people's everyday actions reflect conscious and unconscious knowledge of society and their place in that society. Sociologist Anthony Giddens (1984) explains this as the interplay between practical and discursive consciousness. Practical consciousness is about tacit knowledge and understandings, knowledge that makes it easy for people to go about their lives in their usual social contexts, but that is not easy to articulate. This kind of knowledge is about things that are habitual or routine, such as many aspects of eating. It involves taken-for-granted common sense, and it allows people to act without conscious thought. Discursive consciousness, in contrast, involves knowledge that people can readily put into words. When drawing from it, they can articulate what they are doing and why, offering specific rationalizations. Importantly, both practical and discursive knowledge are shaped by the society in which people live.

The explanations that people provide for their actions reflect the discourses circulating in their society. These discourses, or ways of thinking about an issue or phenomenon, come to define what can be said about something, or even considered possible (Foucault 1979, 1988). Discourses can be produced and circulated by powerful social institutions such as government, universities, industry, and the media, but they are also disseminated, reinforced, resisted, and transformed through people's everyday actions and beliefs (as in Bernice Valverde's description of processed foods as "full of chemicals and colours and additives"). When people articulate rationales for their everyday actions that draw on a certain knowledge, belief, or understanding, that discourse is reinforced, recirculated, and made available to others as reasons for their own behaviour. Thus, the relationship between the knowledge available to people in a society and their actions is reciprocal: people act using socially available knowledge, and their actions inform the knowledge that is readily available.

The habitual, common sense, or unconscious nature of many activities has been explained by French sociologist Pierre Bourdieu (1984) through the concept of *habitus* – the internalized social and cultural influences that shape people's everyday behaviour. Focusing particularly on social class, Bourdieu argues that tastes and preferences learned during early childhood in a specific cultural context become internalized, embodied, unconscious, and part of one's common sense. The social settings of childhood – family, school, friends, piano lessons, hockey practice – evoke particular ways of being and teach particular understandings, tastes, and preferences. Each setting demands certain responses and teaches certain predispositions, which shape how individuals perceive and act in the world, even what foods they like and dislike. Bourdieu helps us to appreciate how individuals are predisposed to act in accordance with the social contexts that shaped them. These dispositions, or tendencies toward particular ways of being, become internalized in the habitus, which can be thought of as the sedimentation of social distinctions (such as class, gender, and ethnicity) within the individual. More concretely, the habitus concept helps us understand why certain eating spaces and foods just *feel* right, whereas others don't. Though one's tastes and preferences are enacted individually, elements are shared by others from the same social location. Thus, for example, both the Valverdes and the Austins emphasized that regularly sitting down together for family meals felt essential for good eating and strong families.

Although Bourdieu's habitus notion is useful, we also know that people have a considerable degree of agency when it comes to culture. There may be group tendencies, but choice remains possible. For example, some lower-income individuals take up French cooking, whereas some higher-class groups eat only fast food. The notion of *cultural repertoires* developed by Ann Swidler (1986) helps us conceptualize how individuals make choices within socially and culturally patterned ways of being. Swidler sees culture not as a monolithic "thing," but as a multi-faceted *set* of skills, habits, styles, and knowledges learned in particular contexts. Individuals acquire a cultural "tool kit," or repertoire of strategies of action based on learned capacities and resources (akin to the set of songs in a musical repertoire). Although people from differing social locations tend to acquire distinct cultural repertoires, they can apply other tools if necessary. They can use numerous elements in their repertoire and can add to it. In many contexts, they draw unconsciously from the repertoire, and they may creatively employ various cultural tools to make sense of the contradictions in their lives and their daily practices. (For example, they may see food in terms of health when they order a salad for lunch but may perceive it as an indulgence when opting for cookies and hot chocolate.) In most everyday settings, people know how to act without thinking about it. It is usually only in unfamiliar settings that they must think about suitable behaviour or consciously learn a new strategy to add to their repertoire. For many people, this rarely occurs, as they gravitate to familiar social settings in which their repertoire provides them with the appropriate cultural tools. However, in times or places of significant adjustment, such as with geographic migration, shifting social or personal circumstances, or periods of rapid social change, people may find themselves more or less consciously going through a period of cultural "retooling," expanding their repertoire to adapt to the new situation.

Swidler's differentiation between conscious and unconscious use of cultural tools provides one example of the relationship between conscious and unconscious influences on actions. French theorist Michel Foucault's ideas regarding the operation of power relations in society are also useful in understanding relationships between conscious and unconscious social actions, as well as how habitual ways of acting can change over time. In contemporary liberal democracies, power commonly functions through discourses, which produce effects by shaping what people do with their bodies, time, and lives (Foucault 1979, 1988). Dominant discourses that establish some foods as good or bad, for example, set up normalizing standards for the behaviour of responsible citizens. As those standards are internalized, they become an ethical or moral compass by which people assess themselves and each other. (Consider Amy Austin's comment, "I would feel like I'm raising them [my family] to be unhealthy if I wasn't preparing their food.") In modern post-industrial societies, force is not normally required to govern a populace; people do the job themselves through a variety of not-always-conscious processes such as surveillance (of self and others), inspection, examination, and confession. These processes simultaneously encourage them to discipline their own behaviour, even as they enable them to present or constitute themselves as good and worthy people.

The multiple discourses in circulation interact in varying ways for people in different social locations. For example, the normalizing standards that define how an upper-middle-class white woman such as Bernice Valverde is expected to behave in Vancouver may differ from the standards internalized by Archie Austin, a teenager in rural Alberta. Both have access to a range of standards (analogous to Swidler's idea of a cultural tool kit), so both can constitute themselves in particular ways to convey certain social identities – as a responsible upper-middle-class mother or as a masculine teenage boy. Social practices such as food habits, then, are not only socially coordinated, but are also performances that convey identity to others (Warde 2005; Halkier 2009; Biltekoff 2013). Certain food practices come to signify who people are and how they wish to portray themselves in terms of social identities. Social categories and distinctions such as gender and class are reproduced or transformed through repeated performances of such practices (Halkier 2009), including those involving food.

In performing their identities, people rely on established distinctions to mark boundaries between social groups. One way of thinking about this is through the concept of "cultural capital," which was developed by Bourdieu (1984). He argues that the tastes, preferences, knowledge, and skills of dominant groups will always be most highly prized and legitimated. People seek to gain such cultural capital to acquire dominance and advantage in a particular social context. This form of capital can consist of knowledge (such as knowing the best kind of vinegar to use in a salad dressing), but it can also take an institutionalized form (such as participating in a class at the prestigious Cordon Bleu school of cooking) or an objectified form (owning an expensive set of Le Creuset pots). To put it simply, the ability to perform, own, or display cultural capital affords higher social status to individuals. Those who cannot display highly valued cultural capital, perhaps because they were raised in a family whose capital was low, may feel a consequent sense of shame and social exclusion, knowing that they do not belong to a high-status cultural grouping. In turn, people may make decisions that are economically unwise but that can bring a sense of belonging, however fleeting, to mainstream consumer society. With regard to food practices, this might occur when people with little money buy highly marketed processed foods that can be seen as symbols of mainstream "normal" consumption, even though public health practitioners and those who hold high cultural capital may frown on such foods as unhealthy and in bad taste (literally and figuratively).

Hierarchies of tastes, where some sets of preferences are more highly prized than others, not only allow people to establish their own identities through social performances, but also to create boundaries between "them" and "us," often with a sense of moral or cultural superiority connected to "us." Sociologist Michèle Lamont (2010, 134) suggests that members of particular socio-cultural groups may share understandings – "cultural scripts concerning what is a worthy person that are partly defined in opposition to scripts perceived to be valued in other groups." Groups construct their own rankings, establishing themselves as worthy on specific grounds in comparison to those who are perceived as higher and lower than themselves. Essentially, though individuals draw boundaries to distinguish themselves, they are also a sign of group membership. The concept of boundary work is vitally important for a study on food because it helps us understand how food consumption defines parameters of inclusion and exclusion across social groupings (see Johnston, Szabo, and Rodney 2011). In other words, deciding to eat a certain food or dine at a certain restaurant is not just about what we feel like eating at a particular moment, but also speaks to who we think we are, which groups we feel a kinship with, and which groups we want to distance ourselves from.

Together, these theoretical approaches form the general framework used to explore and interpret family food practices in the chapters that follow. We view people's eating habits as everyday practices that are moulded by a mix of conscious, semi-conscious, and unconscious influences, many of which are grounded in the social context of their lives. People can explain some aspects of why they eat as they do, drawing on discourses that are available to them in their society. Bernice Valverde, for example, discussed at length why she sometimes chose local, seasonal, conventional produce over imported organic produce, sharing information about the energy used to grow and transport imported or greenhouse crops, as well as the chemicals found in various types of produce. But many food preferences, styles, and decisions reflect internalized norms or understandings that have gotten "under the skin," evoking seemingly automatic strategies of action relating to food. This was illustrated by the Austins, who did not provide a rationale for their traditional frugal approach to eating what the teenagers described as "normal" food that "puts meat on your bones," just as the Valverdes felt no need to explain their adventurous, more costly approach.

Although these families may not be consciously aware of how they acquired these preferred strategies of action or food tastes, sociological analysis suggests that they are a product of – and communicate about – the families' social locations, including aspects of class, gender, ethnicity, and the culture of the places in which they live. A special meal for the Austins involves Amy preparing a feast that reflects their Ukrainian heritage and rural Alberta culture. For the Valverdes, the special meal might be an Indian-themed dinner prepared by Basil and his brother-in-law, both of whom "love to cook," reflecting the cosmopolitan culture of Vancouver and perhaps a particular urban middle-class version of masculinity.

It is particularly important to note that the less-than-fully-conscious influences are not entirely scripted; nor are they immutable. Individuals have a range of behaviours – or, for the purposes of this book, eating styles – that feel comfortable for them in their social contexts. Their repertoire of eating styles will probably change over time as they are exposed to new discourses about food, new environments, and new social groups, or as their own social location and aspirations change. The Austins, for example, have opened their home to a series of Japanese exchange students, with the result that Amy "learned the art of sushi making," and now the whole family loves sushi. Nonetheless, overtones of their traditional tastes remain: according to Amy, they do not like sushi "with raw fish. We like it with crab ... avocado or egg, that type of sushi." But clearly, the Austins' food repertoires have expanded to include a number of items from a variety of ethnic cuisines, other than the typical meat-and-potatoes fare of rural white Canadians.

Some dietary changes may be conscious, as people opt to eat in certain ways in response to new information, beliefs, health issues, or overt social pressures. For example, believing that Bart's growing adolescent body needed meat, Bernice Valverde decided to reintroduce it to the family diet. But other changes may be less conscious, as people observe the behaviours, beliefs, and values demonstrated and communicated by those around them and internalize them as new social standards (such as the Valverdes' enthusiastic embrace of diverse cuisines). People may also resist change, retaining the patterns of childhood, which may no longer fit the social contexts in which they find themselves, resulting in feeling out of place or being seen by others in unfavourable ways.

This points to the relationship between eating practices and identity. What and how people eat communicates to others who they are – what kind of man, woman, parent, or child. Without being fully aware of their actions, people may eat in differing ways in varying social settings because they want to be seen in a certain light by those around them. Identities, as communicated through social performance, are typically not value-neutral, and they are often subject to moral judgment. Certain ways of being are seen by self and others as morally superior, what a "good" person does, whereas other ways of being are seen as irresponsible or lower in status (Biltekoff 2013). Bernice Valverde, for instance, alluded to this kind of hierarchy when she claimed that the diets of the teenagers she knew were not like those of other teens:

> In our social network, I think they're all well-fed, well-exposed kids who get a lot of variety in their diets and try all sorts of different things. Do they eat a typical diet that's making kids obese? I don't think so. I don't think that we fall into that demographic. And I think it is a demographic thing, and it's definitely connected to income and what you were exposed to as a kid.

Bernice went on to talk about the importance of parents being "aware of food issues" and thinking "about where their food comes from." Although she will probably never meet the Austins, one might predict that she would criticize their food practices – that they buy food on sale and, as Anthony stated, are "not too concerned about where it comes from or whether it's organic or anything like that."

Although many everyday practices can shape and convey social identities, food also has a unique place among socio-cultural practices. What we eat is literally incorporated into our bodies, causing physical sensations, responses, and changes. It is experienced through our senses: each dish has a unique combination of scents, tastes, and textures. What we eat affects how we feel, including pleasant sensations of satiation and unpleasant feelings such as excessive fullness, bloating, indigestion, and nausea. We also understand that it has longer-term effects on our bodies. Some of these are visible, such as body size and shape or allergic reactions, whereas others are harder to detect, such as blood sugar or cholesterol levels. These embodied aspects of food are not separate from the social issues considered above, as our experiences and understanding of our bodies are filtered through cultural lenses and cognitive processes. We learn socially what tastes are pleasant and unpleasant, and we also learn that preferences for particular kinds of tastes may distinguish us from others in terms of social hierarchies of class, gender, and ethnicity. And, like "social performances through eating, our sensory experiences of food are deeply embedded in how we express who we are and our relationships with others. What is remarkable is that something so bodily and individual – food – is simultaneously so social.

Despite the rich possibilities offered by the theoretical approach introduced here, in-depth studies that apply it are still much needed. Earlier foundational studies solidly established the understanding that food practices are inherently social and that tastes are collectively constituted. In the United Kingdom, for example, Nickie Charles and Marion Kerr (1988) showed that food consumption could not be extricated from social relations of gender, class, and age, and was central to the construction of particular versions of family. In the United States, Marjorie DeVault's (1991) classic study documented the invisible work of shopping, cooking, and serving meals through which women constructed not just family, but also their identities as women and mothers. In Australia, Deborah Lupton (1996) brought the emphasis more fully back to the body, asking how food was experienced in the body through emotions, tastes, memories, and preferences. Alan Warde's (1997) research productively examined food and taste to explore practices of class, consumption, and consumer behaviour. Most recently, Charlotte Biltekoff (2013) documented how authoritative guidelines and discourses about eating shaped how people understood diet and health, as well as how they saw themselves as good and moral individuals.

This book builds on all these earlier insights, through a study that aims to make sense of people's eating practices while attending to gender, class, and family dynamics, the meanings of consumption patterns, and the embodiment of food practices and taste. More specifically, we explore how social location affects the ways in which people think, talk, and act with respect to food. Similarly, we examine how geographic location – whether people live in a large city, a small town, or a rural area; whether they live in Central Canada, the East

Coast, or Western Canada; whether they have migrated to Canada or moved across it – affects food practices, both through what is or is not available to them locally, and through how other people in the local environment think and talk about food. We examine dominant social discourses about food and eating, but we also ask how people take up, modify, or resist those discourses, according to social and geographic location. Exploring these questions within families allows us to examine how food meanings and habits are formed, transmitted, repelled, and transformed among teens and their parents at the family table.

STUDY DESIGN AND METHODS

To reach these goals, our study employed qualitative social science research methods, with in-depth interviews as the main method of data collection. (For full details about our methods, see Appendix 1.) Participants were recruited from ten Canadian communities, which are described and compared in Table 1. Halifax and Kings County are on the East Coast, in Nova Scotia; Kingston, Prince Edward County, and Toronto's South Parkdale and North Riverdale neighbourhoods are in Central Canada, in Ontario: Edmonton and Athabasca County are in the Prairie region, in Alberta; and Vancouver and the District of Kent are on the West Coast, in British Columbia. Toronto and Vancouver are large, multi-ethnic, cosmopolitan cities; the two Toronto neighbourhoods were chosen to provide contrasts in economic and ethnic diversity within the same city. Edmonton and Halifax are midsized cities, and Kingston is a smaller city. Rural areas, comprised of farms, villages, and small towns, were represented by Kings County, Prince Edward County, Athabasca County, and the District of Kent.

The communities varied in terms of household income, with five having incomes above the 2006 Canadian median of $63,600 (Statistics Canada 2011, 2012). The poorest community was South Parkdale in Toronto, with a median family income of $38,145, whereas the most well-off was Toronto's North Riverdale, with a median family income of $94,204 (City of Toronto 2006a, 2006b). As Table 1 shows, the basic costs of living tended to be higher in the cities than in rural areas, though costs in Nova Scotia were higher than elsewhere except Toronto.

The communities also varied in ethnic diversity. One marker of this is the prominence of people whom Statistics Canada classifies as "visible

TABLE 1 Research Sites

Community	Province (region)	Population[a]	Visible minority (%)[a]	Median family income[a]	Market basket measure[b]	Pseudonym initials
Halifax	Nova Scotia (East Coast)	372,858	7.5	$66,892	$32,303	NH
Kings County	Nova Scotia (East Coast)	47,814	2.0	$48,483–53,254[c]	$31,820	NW
Kingston	Ontario (Central Canada)	152,358	7.1	$67,908	$29,510	KK
Prince Edward County	Ontario (Central Canada)	25,496	1.3	$60,792	$29,221	KC
Toronto (South Parkdale)	Ontario (Central Canada)	2,503,281 (21,005)	"Bit higher" than 46.9[d]	$38,145	$33,177	TP
Toronto (North Riverdale)	Ontario (Central Canada)	2,503,281 (12,430)	"Lower" than 46.9[d]	$94,204	$33,177	TR
Edmonton	Alberta (Prairie)	1,034,935	22.9	$69,214	$31,120	AE
Athabasca County	Alberta (Prairie)	7,587	1.6	$63,270	$30,912	AA
Vancouver	British Columbia (West Coast)	2,116,581	51.0	$58,805	$31,789	BV
District of Kent	British Columbia (West Coast)	4,738	2.9	$51,579	$29,789	BF

a Except for South Parkdale and North Riverdale, data are from Statistics Canada (2011). For South Parkdale and North Riverdale, data are from City of Toronto (2006a, 2006b). For comparison, the 2006 data for Canada as a whole are as follows: population 31,241,030, visible minority 16.2 percent, and median income $63,600.

b Statistics Canada (2013). The market basket measure represents a modest basic standard of living in each location. It includes the costs of food, clothing, footwear, transportation, shelter, and other expenses for a family of two adults and two children.

c Kings County census data are reported separately for four subdivisions. The highest and lowest median family incomes are shown here.

d Specific data for South Parkdale and North Riverdale are not available. The City of Toronto (2006a, 2006b) reported the percentage of visible minority people as a "bit higher" or "lower" than the overall Toronto statistic of 46.9 percent.

minority" (Statistics Canada 2011). In all the rural areas, less than 3 percent of the population consisted of a visible minority. Halifax and Kingston also had quite homogeneous populations, with 7 to 8 percent visible minorities. In Halifax, the most prominent minority is the black African community that has lived there for about four hundred years. In Kingston, the largest visible minority groups are Chinese and South Asian immigrants. Edmonton, with a visible minority population at 23 percent, is somewhat more diverse than Canada as a whole, and Toronto and Vancouver are both highly multicultural, with 47 percent and 51 percent visible minorities respectively. Toronto is arguably the most diverse, with very large Chinese, South Asian, black, and Filipino communities, whereas the Chinese community is clearly the dominant minority group in Vancouver, making up 29 percent of its population.

In all these places, we recruited 9 to 13 families to participate in the study. They had to have lived in the local area for at least two years and had to include at least 1 teenager. "Family" meant whatever it meant to participants, but at least some members were required to live in the household, since we were interested in how people influenced each other. In every family, we interviewed at least 1 teenager (aged thirteen to nineteen) and 1 adult. Across the country, we interviewed members of 105 families, including 123 adults (105 women and 18 men) and 131 youth (77 girls and 54 boys). Among the families, 30 were headed by single mothers, 10 were multi-generational, and 65 included an adult female, an adult male, and 1 or more youth. More detailed demographic information about the sample is provided in Appendix 2.

Each participant was interviewed twice. Interviews were normally conducted separately with each family member, but sometimes teen siblings preferred to be interviewed together, and many of the male parents or guardians preferred to be interviewed with their female partners. In the first interview, which usually lasted one to two hours, people were asked about what they and other members of their family ate; how they decided what to eat; how their eating habits related to their culture, community, and health concerns; and how they made food-related decisions, including who made the decisions and how family members influenced each other.

The second interview probed more deeply into the relationships among place, gender, class, ethnicity, age, and food practices, using two visual research methods to help "get at" the taken-for-granted practical consciousness, or aspects of habitus and cultural repertoires that people may hold instinctually but struggle to articulate. Several scholars suggest that multiple research methods are needed to discern multiple levels of socio-cultural influences on practices (Vaisey 2008; Brown 2009; Silva, Warde, and Wright 2009). Visual photo-elicitation methods, which we used, can be particularly powerful (Power 2003).

After the initial interview, the first photo-elicitation technique was initiated: participants took photographs of foods and eating places in their homes and local community. They were given a list of possible subjects, including foods they did and did not like, foods they ate at home or away from it, places where they would or would not eat out and where they did or did not purchase food, and healthy or unhealthy foods, as well as the interiors of their kitchen cupboards and fridges, if they were willing. If they used the disposable film-based cameras that we supplied, a duplicate set of prints was developed (one for us, one for them to keep) prior to the second interview. Many participants preferred to use their own digital cameras, in which case images were viewed on a computer during the second interview, when we also obtained digital copies. The second interview began with a careful review of the photos, with participants describing them and interviewers asking probing questions.

Although the inclusion of photos taken by participants gave us a good sense of their food worlds, we knew that the exercise would primarily inform us about the foods and ways of eating with which they were comfortable. It would not push them to discuss unfamiliar aspects of food or areas of discomfort. Also, because each participant's set of photos would be unique, comparing the experiences of individuals would be difficult. We therefore included a second photo-elicitation activity, using two sets of stock photographs that we provided. The first set included shots of fifteen types of restaurants, ranging from informal cafeterias and fast-food places to very formal restaurants. We included restaurants that served various types of ethnic cuisines. Participants sorted these photos into piles, indicating where they would feel comfortable eating and where they would not feel comfortable. Some people created a third "neutral" pile. The images were intended to get at a gut-level sense of belonging or not belonging in particular food environments, a sense of comfort or discomfort that might be connected to habitus or cultural repertoires.

The second set of images included twenty-six shots of various foods and meals. We included fast, fancy, and simple foods, foods from various ethnic cuisines, and vegetarian and meat-based meals. Selecting photos of an adequate range of food types, but not making the exercise excessively long, was challenging. It was equally challenging to label them in ways that provided adequate information for the exercise, given the wide range of potential knowledges or cultural repertoires. Participants in large cities or from certain cultural groups might be familiar with many cuisines. Yet people from small towns and rural areas, especially if they hadn't travelled much, might have no idea what some dishes were. Thus, we labelled most typically Euro-Canadian foods by their specific names (beef Wellington, hot dog, grilled cheese sandwich), whereas others were labelled according to their ethnic origin (Korean food, Japanese meal, Ethiopian food, North Indian thali). Not only would many Canadians be entirely unfamiliar with *kimchee, okazu, injera,* or *dhal,* but those photos also included six to twelve dishes in a single meal, making it difficult to name each one. Other "ethnic" foods were labelled more precisely (roti dinner, butter chicken, hummus, falafel, soft-shell tacos).

We asked participants to sort the photos according to which foods they would be comfortable or uncomfortable eating. They also sorted according to whether they thought foods were healthy or unhealthy, adult or teen, typically male or typically female, and whether they were or were not comfortable with preparing them. Again, some people created neutral piles every time. Most importantly, we asked them to talk about *why* they categorized the photos as they did. This activity was designed to overcome challenges noted in our previous research (see Beagan et al. 2008), where direct questions about gender and food were met with silence. The photo-sorting technique was intended to "de-centre the text" (Power 2003), allowing participants to tap knowledges and social rules that might be hard to put into words or awkward to discuss.

Word-for-word transcripts of all the interviews were prepared and entered into a software program (AtlasTi) to help organize our analysis. Key photographs and field notes recording the interviewers' reflections on the interviews were also entered into the software. The main activities of data analysis consisted of reading and rereading transcripts, comparing one person or family with another, comparing patterns by gender, class, place, and ethnicity, and paying attention to people who seemed not to fit in. We collectively developed a list of codes – words to label themes or patterns in the data – such as "tensions" or "cosmopolitanism" or "healthy eating." Once all the data for each family were coded, the analyst wrote a summary "family memo," recording the main themes in the family's food practices. Further analysis for the chapters that follow involved detailed review of specific codes or code combinations, and of the family memos and original transcripts.

Because the research addressed the ways in which social class shapes family food practices, we paid careful attention to how we identified class, which we wanted to be based on the traditional markers of income, education, and employment. In a study based on people's stories rather than survey data, assigning class status was complex. To ensure consistency, we made several key decisions. We assigned class according to household, rather than per individual. Teens were automatically allocated the class status of their parents, since they do not themselves have the traditional markers of class. Where two adults seemed to have differing statuses, we opted for the higher of the two. Our categories focused primarily on occupation (which to some extent incorporates education level and income) and the occupations of the person's parents (how someone grew up). We combined several ways in which class has been defined in the United Kingdom (see Marshall 1998, for the Goldthorpe Typology), the United States (Lamont 1992; Gilbert 2008), France (Bourdieu 1984; Lamont 1992), and Canada (Macionis and Gerber 2011), developing five categories:

1. Upper class: live off existing wealth, top 3–5 percent of the population
2. Upper middle class (high-status white collar): managers, professionals, business people
3. Lower middle class (lower-status white collar, highly skilled blue/pink collar): lower-level administrators and managers, nurses, executive assistants, skilled tradespeople
4. Working class (lower-skilled blue/pink collar): manual and clerical jobs with less formal skills, training, and education
5. Working poor/impoverished: precarious work and insecure incomes that fall at or below the poverty line; reliance on income assistance.

Many families were easy to categorize. In other instances, when education, occupation, and income did not match, or when a family had experienced significant changes in occupation or income over time, we eventually reached consensus after detailed discussion. In most of these hard-to-categorize cases, participants' employment and educational background were consistent with groups 2–4 above, but due to unemployment or disability, they had been living in poverty for some time. Ultimately, we classified these families as "working poor/impoverished" because living in poverty was so dominant in their food practices. We also flagged these (and other) families as having experienced a class trajectory in which they moved from one class to another over time. These families are a focus of Chapter 6. In a few families, the adults did manual labour but ran small businesses to provide it; we categorized them as lower middle class.

Throughout the study, we were attentive to ethical aspects of research practice. The research was reviewed and approved by ethics boards at the five universities where we were employed. All adult participants provided informed consent. For interviewees who were under the age of consent, their assent and parental consent were obtained. Because of the intersectional nature of our analysis, we reveal some demographic details regarding participants but have done our best to remove identifying information: all names are pseudonyms, and some details such as occupations have been changed (though always remaining in the same class category). Participants in any given site were assigned names that began with the same letters. So, for example, all British Columbians who lived in Vancouver, such as Bernice Valverde, were assigned the initials BV. Interviewees who lived in Alberta's Athabasca County, such as Amy Austin, were given the initials AA. Using this scheme meant that everyone's geographic location could immediately be discerned from their names. The pseudonym initials are listed in Table 1.

Like class, ethnicity is notoriously difficult to define. We have provided the age, ethnicity, and class of all participants whom we quote in this book. We asked people to self-identify in terms of ethnicity. Generally, however, dominant social groups (such as white-skinned Canadians of European heritage) don't tend to see themselves as members of a group at all. They are just "Canadian." Yet we know that race and ethnicity make a difference to people's experiences. So, for those participants of white European heritage who were born in Canada and simply called themselves Canadian, we used the label "white." This is an imperfect category. For individuals who were born in Europe and who self-identified as, for example, British or German, we used that label. Thus, someone who moved to Canada from Germany would be a "German Canadian," whereas someone whose grand-parents immigrated from Germany was simply described as "white." In this scheme, people with vastly different ethnic heritages, and vastly different relationships to their heritages, are lumped together as "white," yet the approach also recognizes the power of white-skinned privilege. Whiteness is not all the same, but white Canadians do collectively experience an advantage that their darker-skinned counterparts do not share. We used the term "white" in recognition of this unearned (and often unintended) advantage.

Also, in terms of ethnicity, it is worth noting that we chose not to study an Aboriginal community. Some Aboriginal families did participate, especially in the cities, but we did not specifically select an Aboriginal study site. Given the unique situation of Aboriginal peoples – the distinctive history of colonialism, the ongoing racism, treaty rights and negotiations, land claims, legal battles over food procurement, displacement from traditional lands, and widespread government-supported conditions of poverty – contemporary Aboriginal food practices warrant their own independent study. There are excellent Aboriginal (and non-Aboriginal) scholars embarked on exactly that research (see, for example, Boult 2004; Ferguson 2011; Martin 2011).

Finally, as feminist scholars, we want to acknowledge our own position as white, upper-middle-class, urban-living women researchers. The task of making sense of practice, exploring how ways of eating are based in the material and cultural aspects of people's lives, can be especially challenging when the analyst's (or reader's) class location or logic of practice differ from those of the subjects. The usual unreflexive tendency is to impose the analyst's logic and unwritten rules of social practice on research participants, which often results in judging their practices as inferior, thus potentially causing harm. Our study method called for rigorous reflexivity to constantly question and account for the distance between our own social positions and those of participants, and to understand the logics of their practices, even (and especially) when it was hard to agree with or condone them.

OVERVIEW OF THE BOOK

In the following chapters, we draw on interview data gathered across Canada to examine in depth how social and cultural factors influence food practices in families. We attend to the ways in which food practices are influenced by gender, social class, race, ethnicity, age, and family roles. We explore the ways in which people are affected by deeply engrained, unconscious, or semi-conscious approaches to food, and how they interact with and use discourses about food in more conscious ways. We also scrutinize how these social and cultural influences may differ by geographic place, in cities or small towns, in one neighbourhood or another, on the East Coast or the West Coast. Cultural repertoires are shaped by local culture, and the discourses that circulate concerning food are at least partially moulded by the local environment.

The first three chapters lay out prominent discourses regarding food practices and beliefs, showing how they connect to gender, class, and place. Chapter 1 takes up one of the most influential contemporary normative discourses concerning food – healthy eating. This is promoted everywhere – in magazines, on television, through schools and health care providers, and on food packaging. People have no choice but to engage with this institutionally sanctioned discourse. Chapters 2 and 3 discuss more emergent food discourses. Chapter 2 deals with ethical eating, a relatively recent subject for the mainstream media and one that has tentative institutional support. Yet it is obviously expanding (even Tim Hortons has begun to promote a fair-trade coffee).* We ask how engagement with ethical eating is shaped by class and place.

Cosmopolitan eating (Chapter 3) is the most implicit of the three discourses. It prizes breadth and variety across cuisines from many ethnicities and is evident in the food sections of newspapers, on television food shows, and in cookbooks. When fast-food restaurants add chipotle chicken to their menus, and gas station diners put Thai chili

. . . .

* For more information on the Tim Hortons Coffee Partnership, the stated intent of which "is to improve the lives of small-scale coffee farmers by increasing the productivity of their farms and the quality of their beans in an environmentally sustainable way," see http://www.timhortons.com/ca/en/difference/coffee-partnership.html.

sauce on the table with the ketchup, cosmopolitan eating is gaining ground. News headlines may not exhort people to engage in it, as is the case with healthy eating, but it is clearly becoming an important way of thinking and talking about food that shapes and is shaped by people's everyday practices.

Chapters 4 through 8 centre on family, gender, class, and place. They ask how these social factors shape food practices, but they also ask how food practices are used to simultaneously *construct* family, gender, class, and place. Chapter 4, on vegetarian eating, focuses on *family* dynamics and highlights a unique aspect of our study – the inclusion of interviews with teens. In part, it examines how the discourses of healthy and ethical eating are applied in family contexts and how they are affected by social class. Chapter 5, on body image, keeps the spotlight on teens, but concentrates on *gender* and its intersection with healthy eating. It shows that though eating for weight loss remains overwhelmingly the purview of women and girls, teen boys may also adopt it under the guise of healthy eating. The chapter reveals that a dominant discourse, such as healthy eating, can expand its reach in numerous directions, even challenging gender norms for food consumption.

The following three chapters scrutinize change, and resistance to it, when the social, cultural, and/or geographic context is altered. Chapter 6 brings the theme of *class* to the fore, exploring food practices and tensions in families where the financial situation of one or more members differs significantly from that of their upbringing. Here we specifically examine how the discourses of healthy, ethical, and cosmopolitan eating may be used to convey particular messages about belonging in terms of class. Chapters 7 and 8 centre on the theme of *place*. The first explores food practices among those who have moved within Canada, particularly how they use talk about food to draw boundaries between self and Other. We found that participants referred more often to rural-urban distinctions than to regional differences. They constructed images of rural and urban ways of eating – and of rural and urban people – by talking about local food practices as healthy (or not), ethical (or not), and cosmopolitan (or not). Chapter 8 looks at eating practices and food-related identities when place is disrupted through migration to Canada from elsewhere. Relationships between ethnicity and place are clearly central here, but equally critical are the ways in which ethnocultural identity intersects with gender expectations and generational differences in families.

Chapter 9 brings everything full circle, asking how food preferences and distinctions, which feel so thoroughly individual and are so thoroughly embodied, are created through social processes in families. In the book as a whole, we argue that food practices are never solely individual, resting on personal tastes, preferences, and bodily reactions. Our empirical data show that social discourses about food not only shape everyday eating in families, but also become part of how people construct and convey their social and cultural identities. Food is inextricably social, affected by and affecting social categories and hierarchies. In Chapter 9, we return to the individual self through embodied sensations. We explore how social rules, tastes, and distinctions become embodied through culturally informed everyday sensory experiences. The chapter inevitably returns to the family, with all its distinct gendered roles in cultural groups, asking how families teach the very food tastes that are used in so many ways to distinguish social groups.

Through food practices learned at the family table, people enact class, place, and gender. Social class forms food practices in ways that reach far beyond the mere availability of resources. To put it bluntly, this study shows that poverty and lack of resources make it very difficult to eat with dignity. For participants who lived in poverty, following the dictates of healthy eating was a significant challenge, and pursuing other food-related practices that can indicate higher social status, such as ethical and cosmopolitan eating, was even more difficult. Geographic place also made certain ways of eating more or less readily available, and customary, with the result that urban food practices were seen as sophisticated and righteous, whereas their rural equivalents were imagined as backward, unsophisticated, unhealthy, traditional, and bland. Though migrants to Canada were least engaged with mainstream discourses about food, they were influenced by gender and their own relationships to ethnic and national identities, and had adjusted their eating practices accordingly. Gender was centrally implicated in engagement with healthy eating and with body image projects. Many adult female participants constructed self-identities, subject positionings, as "good mothers" in part through ensuring healthy eating at the family table.

Relationships to food and food discourses were widely used, not only to construct the self, but also to judge the Other. This study shows that notions of healthy, ethical, and cosmopolitan eating are not morally or socially neutral. In drawing on, transforming, resisting, or rejecting them, people's everyday eating creates and maintains deep, inequitable social divisions on the basis of class, place, and gender. When people engage with food, there is a lot going on beneath the surface – thus, changing eating practices is socially and morally fraught. Eating is not solely about fuelling the body: it is also about conveying to self and others particular social identities and positions in numerous social hierarchies.

1

healthy eating

The Fagan Family

THE FAGAN FAMILY lives in the District of Kent, in British Columbia's Fraser Valley. Bree Fagan (fifty-six) is an alternative health practitioner, and her husband, Boyd (fifty-nine), is a chef, though at the time of our interviews, he was on leave from his job due to a stroke some months earlier. The Fagans, who are white and of European heritage, have an annual household income of $50,000 to $75,000. Their two oldest children have left home, and their daughter Beata (sixteen) is finishing high school.

Healthy eating is very important to the Fagans. Boyd and Bree agree that it is their top priority in food choice, with taste and convenience much lower priorities. As Bree says, "Taste might not be that important if you know that [less tasty food] is going to keep you healthy. Taste is just a habit." They started eating almost exclusively organic food about twenty-five years earlier, "before it became mainstream." Although they have strong views on ethics and the politics of food production and consumption, their primary motivation is health. They prepare everything from scratch, even making their own almond milk.

According to Bree, "It basically all started because of health issues." In the past, she had multiple undiagnosed ailments, which she now thinks were "fibromyalgia and chronic fatigue and hypoglycemia and so on." In response to this, Bree says, "We started taking health not for granted any more and started working with it and looking at what can we do to stay well and be healthy." Assuming that she had food allergies, they began a very restricted elimination diet, gradually reintroducing foods to determine which ones caused symptoms. For years, they rotated "safe" foods to allow their immune systems to recover.

The Fagans believe that Bree has "sensitivities to wheat and milk, and sugar was a big culprit too." They feel that learning about nutrition to safeguard their health is their responsibility. Bree argues that attention to diet has "totally" restored her health and notes that food sensitivities have also affected the children: "Wheat and milk were culprits with our older one too, also processed foods, food colourings, flavourings, preservatives, sugars." Their son was hyperactive and had "pounding headaches, cramps in his legs, tummy upset, and earaches." These disappeared with dietary change. Bree also states that her daughter had "personality changes" when she ate the "wrong" foods: "She would be like another person." The Fagans carefully control what their children eat, to the point of picking them up from birthday parties before cake is served so they don't eat it. Boyd hinted that this is sometimes difficult: "So many times we had to say no. You can't have this, you can't have that. It's hard for kids."

Boyd and Bree prioritize what they consider healthy eating, even when such choices are more expensive: "Definitely healthy comes over cost ... We spend probably a third more, at least, buying organic and trying to live healthy." Both Bree and daughter Beata note that they have immediate physical reactions to foods that were sprayed with chemicals. Beata admitted that she sometimes indulges in chocolate even though her face breaks out: "That's my responsibility. It's my body. I choose to eat it." Generally, though, she prefers to eat well: "I like eating healthy food because it makes me feel better, plain and simple. I just feel better when I eat well."

Despite decades of healthy eating, Boyd had a stroke some months before our interview. This caused him some uncertainty concerning their diet: "I always felt that we were eating healthy, compared to mainstream. Which we probably did. And it still hit me." He attributes his stroke to stress, whereas Bree suggests that he ate less well at work than at home. Since his stroke, the Fagans have intensified healthy eating, using diet to lower Boyd's already low cholesterol. He eats more fish and nuts, and starts the day with a "green smoothie" composed of juice, algae, kale, Swiss chard, celery, cucumber, and apple.

Boyd hinted at some of the difficulties of maintaining such rigorous healthy eating, mentioning that the Fagans are somewhat marginalized socially: "Food is such a big part of life. So it's not easy to do it, because it also isolates you socially. People tend not to invite you any more. 'Well what should we cook for them?' ... People are not comfortable." In turn, the Fagans speak somewhat harshly about those who "choose not to take responsibility" for healthy eating. They believe that those who smoke, drink, or eat sweets could easily afford to feed their family healthfully, if they were willing "to prioritize." Bree acknowledges that their approach to food is not centred on pleasure, stating, "If eating and food is all you can do for fun, then I feel sorry for you."

Overall, the Fagans stand out – in both their own community and our study – for their strong commitment to healthy eating and their relatively restrictive approach.

· · · *The Wood Family*

THE WOOD FAMILY, which is white and upper middle class, lives in Kings County, Nova Scotia, and has a household income of about $140,000. Nigel (forty-five) is in the Armed Forces. His daughters Nadia (seventeen) and Nallely (fifteen) are in high school. His wife, Nanette (forty-three), the girls' stepmother, is an employment counsellor. For the Woods, any hint of dietary restriction is strenuously resisted. Their priorities are taste and convenience, with nutrition a distant third.

All the Woods describe healthy eating as centring on vegetables. Nanette emphasizes salads, and Nadia and Nallely stress the importance of whole grains, fruit juices, and soy milk. The teens believe that the family generally eats healthfully, primarily due to their father. Nigel makes an effort to eat vegetables, as an example for his daughters, but Nanette dislikes cooked vegetables and refuses to eat them. Nigel comments,

> I could go without vegetables for quite a bit. You give me a roast chicken, mashed potatoes, I'm good. But okay, there should be something green on the plate. So we make sure we have frozen vegetables on hand to make some for the kids. And then I eat some to set a good example. Someone

else at the table here doesn't eat the vegetables often, but I do, just to set a good example.

In defining "unhealthy" foods, the Woods emphasize fast foods, especially McDonald's and KFC, chips, pop, pizza, white bread, cookies, cakes, and sugary cereals. Nigel and Nanette added salt, sugar, and fat to the list, especially trans fats. When asked what the effects of unhealthy eating might be, all four mentioned weight gain, with Nigel adding decreased longevity and his daughters citing heart disease. Nallely referred to fast food as a "heart attack waiting to happen" and as something to be eaten rarely. Nigel and Nanette, however, eat at McDonald's fairly regularly: "Our guilty pleasure."

According to Nanette, the family sometimes strives to eat healthfully but sabotages its own efforts:

> We were making a really healthy meal ... We got chicken and we got lettuce and we got wraps and all that stuff, and then we decided we needed bacon ... So that's an entire pound of bacon cooking up into little bits that we put all over our thing. So we have good intentions and then we sabotage them ... We had to bread the chicken and then fry it before we put it in our Caesar wrap.

According to Nigel, healthy eating messages are everywhere: "I couldn't say where I learned, like, I just know." He was introduced to Canada's Food Guide at school, and his parents taught him about healthy eating. He says, "It's just common sense; I mean if you're not stupid, you can figure it out." Nallely and Nadia also encounter consistent messages about healthy eating through school, their parents, and "word of mouth – everyone's." Nadia recalls "those really annoying lectures that your teachers give you from the fourth grade onward about how important healthy eating is. It gets to the point where you're just, like, 'We know already. Teach us something else!'"

The adult Woods clearly understand healthy eating messages but frequently resist them – both deliberately and subconsciously, as when Nanette describes sabotaging their Caesar wraps with bacon. Nigel sees himself as lucky that he has never gained weight, claiming that his body is naturally "self-regulating." Consequently, he has never paid serious attention to health or nutrition and wouldn't do so unless he were advised by a doctor to lose weight. He rejects healthy eating messages, insisting that pleasure is more valuable than longevity. Nigel insists that he would rather enjoy a shorter life than extend his time through an unenjoyable regimen, which he terms "going to an extreme." In fact, both Nigel and Nanette spoke rather scornfully about others whom they see as overly obsessed with nutrition, including Nigel's vegetarian brother, whom they describe as "kind of sickly" looking. According to Nigel, "He actually looks too thin ... He doesn't enjoy his food." Nanette added, "He exercises, like, a whole lot ... He's really careful about every single thing he puts in his body. He doesn't look like he has a whole lot of fun."

Not only does Nigel perceive "extremes" of healthy eating to be dangerous, but he hinted that non-organic foods might be good for people, suggesting that pesticides "really aren't that bad" and could even contribute to "people living longer, healthier lives than they ever have in the history of the world."

The Wood family, in sum, clearly understands "common sense" messages about healthy eating and feels slight guilt about not following them more fully, but mostly believes that healthy eating hinders the enjoyment of food. The Woods are unconvinced that healthy eating is wholly desirable and bristle at the idea of food restrictions and reduced pleasures in the interest of health.

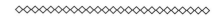

THE NOTION OF "healthy eating" was ubiquitous in our conversations with families. We ourselves wanted to explore the issue, but it was also a core part of how most study participants thought and spoke about food. They spontaneously described foods as healthy or unhealthy, or talked about their own ways of eating in those terms.* When asked about healthy eating, they rarely sought clarification. Everyone understood the concept that food affects health, both positively and negatively, and it figured centrally in their evaluation of their own and others' eating habits. It also appeared to shape negotiations and decisions about what to eat.

* Throughout this chapter, "healthy" and "unhealthy" refer to the ideas of participants, not to our own judgments regarding foods or eating patterns. In addition, "masculine" and "feminine," as applied to food, are constructs for analysis; we do not suggest that food is inherently gendered or that it should be.

But participants were just as likely to discuss how they did *not* meet the healthy eating ideal. It was a kind of "gold standard" that virtually no one fully attained. Some felt guilty about this, whereas others laughed it off. Some tried to encourage family members to eat "healthier," and some resisted this pressure. Notions of healthy eating played a powerful role in determining how participants ate, but people also used these concepts – engaging with and resisting them – to convey critical ideas about their identities. The case studies above, for example, contrast the Fagans' presentation of themselves as highly responsible, self-regulating individuals who were perhaps morally superior to many people they knew, with the Woods' identity as pleasure-focused, fun-loving people.

THEORETICAL FRAMING

The concept of discourse, as understood by Michel Foucault and others who built on his work, is fundamental to our examination of healthy eating. For Foucault (1979, 1980), discourses are the ways of understanding a phenomenon that circulate through a society. Dominant discourses are supported by major social institutions such as governments and educational systems, and by the authority of "expert" knowledge. In contemporary societies, knowledge produced through science may be valued more highly than other kinds of knowledge (such as anecdotal observation, intuition, or tradition). Discourses that are validated through scientific research enjoy strong social and institutional support, which is also gained through endorsement by experts such as scientists, doctors, and university professors (like the authors of this book!). These are not the only sources of support for discourses, however. They are in continual circulation through society, with various forms of media being perhaps the most obvious venue. They are also disseminated through everyday interactions, such as through conversations, observing the actions of others, and self-monitoring.

For any given phenomenon, multiple discourses, or ways of understanding, will be in play at any given time. Views that are most widely distributed – that are consistently promoted by major social institutions, by experts, in the media, and through everyday interactions – constitute dominant discourses. Other understandings may be marginal and can cohere to form oppositional discourses. As discourses continue to circulate, shifts occur, with some understandings gaining credence and others falling out of favour. For example, as increasing numbers of people embrace a marginal discourse, and as it receives broader circulation and visibility through the media, it gains strength and may eventually be incorporated into or become the dominant discourse. Discourses are thus continually changing, and people's everyday actions and conversations are part of this. When people speak and act in ways that are consistent with a discourse, they reinforce and reinscribe it. When their actions oppose it, they diminish its strength and create or reinforce an oppositional discourse that may eventually supplant it.

Foucault viewed discourse as inextricably linked with power. Much of his writing details the ways in which discourses produce effects through organizing people's activities, time, movement, and thoughts. His notion of "governmentality" – the ways in which the behaviour of populations, societies, and institutions are governed or directed – expands on the relationship between discourse and power (Foucault 1991). Where once it may have been acceptable to control or govern a population with physical force, more subtle forms of regulation are required in liberal democratic societies (Foucault 1979; Power forthcoming). Discourses set social standards governing behaviour, thus regulating people. Supported by social institutions, dominant discourses define the ways in which "good citizens" should behave.

Current neoliberal political climates strongly emphasize that individuals must take responsibility for acting in socially accountable ways, demonstrating themselves to be moral, virtuous citizens (Coveney 1999, 2000). This is perhaps nowhere clearer than in relation to health: people are expected to pursue it actively, and "personal responsibility for health is widely considered the *sine qua non* of individual autonomy and good citizenship" (Crawford 2006, 402). This pressure is intensified in the Canadian context of publicly funded health care, where behaviours that increase health risks can be viewed as a drain on health care dollars. Yet there is evidence that, for well over a century, nutritional science has served to govern people through insisting on personal responsibility for dietary health; discourses about food provide one way for people to display their own moral character (Biltekoff 2013).

This relationship between discourse and individuals' demonstration of themselves as good people raises another key point: the role of discourse in the constitution of the self, or identity. Identity is not a fixed entity. Instead, it is continually formed, demonstrated, and reformed within discourse. Because discourses are multiple and shifting, people may position themselves in relation to differing discourses to portray themselves in various ways, processes that Foucault (1988) refers to as "technologies of the self." Other scholars have pointed out that discourses are gendered, classed, racialized, and so on (Weedon 1987; Bordo 1993; Bartky 1997; Biltekoff 2013). The discourses that are most available to, or dominant, for women of certain classes or races differ markedly from those that are available to men or women in other social locations. Thus, men and women in differing social locations may relate to discourses quite differently as they strive to present themselves as good or moral, responsible people. Similarly, dominant discourses are specific to time and place, so they may vary by time and geographic location.

PARTICIPANTS, PLACES, AND APPROACH TO ANALYSIS

This chapter focuses on participants from four communities: Vancouver and the District of Kent in British Columbia and Halifax and Kings County in Nova Scotia. A large, ethnically diverse city, Vancouver is relatively young, whereas Halifax is a mid-sized city whose roots stretch back to the seventeen hundreds. Its people are predominantly of English, Irish, and Scottish heritage. The District of Kent and Kings County are smaller, more rural areas, with predominantly white Euro-Canadian populations scattered on farms and in small towns and villages.

The eleven Vancouver families who participated in our study lived in a relatively low-income area but had a range of incomes. About half identified as Euro-Canadian, and the rest defined their heritage as Aboriginal, South Asian, Chinese, or "other." The income levels in the Halifax sample also covered the full range, and its ten families were mostly Euro-Canadian, with a few Aboriginal and African-heritage participants. In the District of Kent, the eleven families tended to be lower middle class and low income, with one upper-middle-class family. Almost all were white and Euro-Canadian. The ten Kings County families were similar; most were working class and working poor, and a few were middle class. All were of Euro-Canadian heritage.

The data analyzed for this chapter included interviews with fifty-two adults and fifty-one teens. The analysis focused on interview comments regarding healthy or unhealthy foods, how subjects understood healthy or unhealthy eating, where they got information about the subject, and their own habits or goals concerning health and eating. Interviews with women, men, girls, and boys were reviewed separately to identify gender and age trends. In addition, we wrote summaries to identify how healthy eating was addressed in each family as a unit. Finally, the interview data and the family summaries were compared across the four locations, to explore any systematic differences by place.

HEALTHY EATING DISCOURSES

When asked what healthy meant to him, Barrett Vale, a sixteen-year-old, white, and lower-middle-class El Salvadoran Canadian, replied:

> What does healthy eating mean to me? I guess getting all your vitamins and nutrients, and just staying healthy and active. I would put it under the category of eating right ... I think of fruits and vegetables and fresh meats, and I just think of fresh. So you know, try to watch calories and whatever people watch nowadays. I don't know, fats, calories, sugars. It's always changing. But yeah, you know, fresh fruits and vegetables and getting all of your greens.

Study participants were largely consistent in defining "healthy" and "unhealthy" eating, both when asked directly and through spontaneous comments. As was evident in the Wood family above, vegetables (especially salads), fruits, whole grains, legumes, low-fat milk, yoghurt, fish, and poultry were commonly described as healthy, and healthy eating was seen as involving variety and "the four food groups." Participants also mentioned the importance of fresh, whole, or unprocessed items, and of foods that provide essential nutrients, such as protein, vitamins, and minerals. Unhealthy eating, in contrast, was generally agreed to involve "junk foods" such as candy, potato chips, ice cream, soft drinks, white bread, and hot dogs. More broadly, foods that are high in fat, sugar, salt, and (less commonly) alcohol and caffeine were perceived as unhealthy. Processed and fried foods, and eating too much also fell into this category.

Almost all participants, regardless of gender, age, or location, talked about healthy and unhealthy eating in this manner, revealing the ascendancy of what can be considered a "mainstream" or dominant healthy eating discourse (Chapman and Beagan 2003; Ristovski-Slijepcevic, Chapman, and Beagan 2008). Linked with official institutions such as governments, universities, and health associations, this discourse circulates broadly through various media (Biltekoff 2013). Canada's Food Guide (mentioned by Nigel Wood as having taught him about healthy eating) is an example of this. Since 1942, the federal government has provided guidance to translate nutritional science into advice to help Canadians choose foods that promote health (Health Canada 2007). Like the mainstream healthy eating discourse of which it is a part, the food guide gains authority from its basis in scientific evidence. The discourse, illustrated in Barrett Vale's comments above, employs the scientific approach in referring to food components such as fats and calories.

Though associated with science and governments, dominant discourses are also promoted and dispersed throughout society more accessibly. Some participants learned about healthy eating through schools, as was the case for Nigel Wood and his daughter Nadia. Others learned from doctors or dietitians, often in relation to particular health issues. For example, Bernadette Vickers (thirty-nine, Native and Irish Canadian, working poor/impoverished) learned about the four food groups from a nutritionist when she was pregnant: "I wasn't putting on enough weight, so they told me how much I should be eating." Participants also learned from books, magazines, and pamphlets. As Nuala Haldane (forty, white, working class) said, "just general reading about healthy eating ... books, magazines, the health books at work." Many had difficulty explaining how they had learned about the subject. Dominant discourses spread widely through informal channels, often in the context of everyday social relationships. People had learned about healthy eating from their mothers and their friends. As Nallely Wood commented, she had learned about nutrition through "word of mouth – everyone's." Mainstream notions of healthy eating were considered taken for granted and common sense.

Despite the prominence of this discourse, some families voiced different understandings of healthy eating, which is not surprising, as discourses are continually changing. One variation (which might be considered a traditional discourse) emphasized homemade, whole foods and traditional meal patterns. This was exemplified by Nicola Weaver (thirty-three, white, working poor/impoverished), for whom healthy eating meant, "I'd like everybody to have milk. I'd like everybody to have meat and vegetables, when I think healthy. Like, they're sitting down and they're having their meat and vegetables and not having things precooked." Nola Wheeler (fifty, white, working poor/impoverished) had a similar outlook:

> It's not something like those TV dinners ... It's a meal that is pre-pared, so it's mostly then going to be from fresh food that, like, you cooked the meat. It's not meat that's prepackaged or with a lot of chemicals type of thing. I don't think it matters about fat content ... It's the processed food that I think is a problem, even if it's diet [food] – processed food, I just don't think the body was meant to eat that stuff.

A traditional healthy eating discourse is distinguished by its emphasis on natural unprocessed foods, home cooking, and meals consisting of meat and vegetables, as well as indifference to nutritional components or food properties. Participants who subscribed to this view tended to engage less than others with healthy eating discussions. Unlike its mainstream counterpart, the traditional discourse came primarily from personal experience and family.

The other main variant on healthy eating was an "alternative" dis-course, mostly espoused by interviewees who were highly engaged in healthy eating efforts, concerned about harmful components in foods, and mistrustful of dominant nutrition messages. The Fagan family fits this description, with its absolute prioritization of healthy eating and its strict control of food choices. For many years, the Fagans closely regulated what they and their children ate, avoiding items that they considered highly toxic, such as artificial colours, preservatives, and sugar. For them, healthy eating included a variety of nutritional sup-plements, algae smoothies, and exclusively organic produce. Despite Boyd Fagan's recent stroke, they strongly believed that healthy eating could ensure good health. They also thought that foods had immedi-ate effects on how they felt physically, as well as on behaviour, mood, and appearance.

The alternative discourse was also predominant for Beatrice Valeriani (fifty-three, Italian and Native, working poor/impoverished), who had recently returned to a raw food diet:

> Because of my energy levels and this weight problem, my inability to digest cooked foods very well, I started on the raw foods again. It's the green drinks, and then you can do all kinds of things. You use a lot of nuts and seeds ... You get a lot of nutrition – tremendous nutrition – when it's not cooked. That's why it has so much nutrition in it. And a lot of people are real die-hard vegetarians, but for myself – my naturopath agrees, he says, "Have a piece of chicken now and again. Have some fish, have a piece of protein."

Both the traditional and the alternative discourse promoted natural unprocessed foods. However, proponents of the traditional approach appeared to value it because it had been practised for generations, whereas those who favoured the alternative discourse were much more specific about why natural foods were superior. They were highly suspicious of additives in processed foods and of environmental contamination, monoculture, and factory farming. Newlyn Henderson (thirteen, white, upper middle class), for example, thought the free-range, organic meat that her parents bought was healthier than conventional meat "because there's not all those steroids and stuff in it; I guess your body would digest them, but the toxins would be in your body." Such toxins were seen as causing immediate and long-term negative effects such as indigestion, allergies, and cancer. As Brett Vessey (fifty-three, British Canadian, upper middle class) said, "With the cancer rates and so on, I just think there's so much chemicals in everything that we do, you know, from breathing air to ingesting food. I think we're healthier if we stay away from the chemicals that are put into foods." Beatrice Valeriani graphically described the harms of typical contemporary diets:

> If you're eating a lot of bread and pizzas and cheeses, lot of meats, and you can't push that through your intestines fast enough, you can get cancer in your colon; you can have troubles with your liver because it's accumulating all the fat and the toxins, and your

body begins to swell up due to the allergies from the foods that you're eating.

The fact that [milk] is pasteurized, it's homogenized, it's dead, there are no enzymes in it, we can't digest it. So children have all kinds of problems, colds and flus and snot running down their face, and that's all from milk. And meat, we know they're getting antibiotics and stuff, and it's even making us have more moles ... 'cause we're eating the hormones and the antibiotics.

The alternative discourse also promoted natural foods and nutritional supplements, such as the Fagan family's "green smoothies." Similarly, Belinda Veitch (forty-nine, Scottish and First Nations, working poor/impoverished) suggested that garlic had medicinal, anti-bacterial, anti-viral properties and described "a whole dietary and vitamin regime that you can use for Alzheimer's as well. Coenzyme Q10 and Vitamin E is right up there, also ... fish oils, flax seed oil." As in the mainstream discourse, foods are seen as comprised of nutrients and other components that have specific health effects.

Beatrice Valeriani's reference to her naturopath illustrates another characteristic of the alternative discourse. Unlike its mainstream counterpart, which is promoted by dominant institutions, it is endorsed by the complementary/alternative medical system and counterculture food and health industries. Participants had learned about healthy eating from naturopaths, other alternative health practitioners, health food stores, books, magazines, and nutritional supplement literature. Beatrice Valeriani, arguably the strongest proponent of the alternative approach, saw health and eating as mystical and spiritual. She was highly skeptical of the dominant discourse, arguing that it was manipulated by institutional interests: "It's a corporate-fed system where big money is ruling."

In sum, though everyone was familiar with notions of healthy eating, understandings of the topic and sources of information differed. Participants who were aligned with the alternative discourse tended to be most strongly engaged in healthy eating efforts and took considerable personal responsibility for learning about nutrition, their bodies, and their health, whereas traditionalists had the least to say about healthy eating. It is important to note that though some participants espoused just one discourse – such as the Fagans – others drew on more than one as they described healthy eating. Barrett Vale, for example, whose quote at the beginning of this section typifies mainstream understandings, also employed an alternative discourse when he spoke about a cleansing fast he had done and that his mother did regularly: "It cleanses your body of toxins and such ... It's a healthy thing to do every once in a while. If you're, like, feeling gross or icky or whatever, just go on a juice fast. It's amazing what it does ... It's, like, scientific or something."

When we examined the interviews by place to determine whether geographic location affected how people thought and talked about healthy eating, we found that the mainstream approach dominated in all four sites. Though the traditional and alternative discourses appeared in every site, the former was more obvious in Nova Scotia and, to a lesser extent, in rural British Columbia, whereas the latter seemed to be strongest in British Columbia (particularly Vancouver). This may relate to the history and demographics of the communities. The Nova Scotia sites are relatively homogeneous in terms of culture, with longer history of settlement, little impact of recent immigration, and longer family history in one place, all of which may reinforce valuing traditional ways of life. Vancouver, in contrast, is highly diverse, with significant mixing of people from various parts of Canada and the world, all of which may support openness to alternative ways of thinking (Ristovski-Slijepcevic, Chapman, and Beagan 2008). As we discuss below, however, though participants' understanding and use of healthy eating discourses may relate in some ways to where they live, shop, and eat, they are more obviously linked to other aspects of identity and sense of self.

GOVERNMENTALITY AND THE MORALITY OF HEALTHY EATING

Discourses entail more than ways of understanding, and those of participants encompassed much more than knowledge or beliefs about healthy eating. Healthy eating discourses clearly set social standards that interviewees used to judge themselves and others, and to support their identities as good people. Some proudly presented themselves as very healthy eaters, whereas others were satisfied with striking a balance between healthy eating and pleasure and cost. Some acknowledged that their diets were not very healthy, and though this admission often involved guilt or inadequacy, a few presented it positively, as a way of opposing the pervasive privileging of personal responsibility for health.

Many participants believed that people have an individual responsibility to eat healthfully, perhaps none more so than the Fagan family. Bree Fagan stated several times that people must take personal responsibility for what they eat and for their own health. She and her husband, Boyd, consistently enacted their convictions, prioritizing health over cost and convenience, and willingly sacrificing taste. The Fagans drew a symbolic boundary between themselves and those who were less committed to the goal of healthy eating. Bree noted that "we are a little different from many people" in this regard, and she took pride in her ability to refuse "unhealthy" foods, saying "it's knowledge and it's dedication that gets me through." Her daughter Beata (sixteen) was similarly proud of the family's healthy eating practices, saying, "I think it's really good that we eat so much vegetables and fruit," and turning up her nose as she talked about a friend's family where "there's never any fruit or vegetables or anything ... Eww!"

Other participants also presented themselves as virtuous or moral individuals as they differentiated between their eating habits and those of other people. This implied that some foods were more sophisticated than others, but it also imputed a lesser moral status to those who ate low-brow and unhealthy food. This often occurred when people described their impressions of other people's choices in a grocery store. For example, Bess Forwell (fifty-four, British Canadian, lower middle class) and her husband, Brendan (forty-six, German Canadian, lower middle class), described themselves as "snobs" and "a bit disdainful" of people who bought "big packages of bologna and Kraft Dinner in the club case pack," "flats of pop, flats of cheap white bread," and "a six pack of Cheez Whiz and condiments galore." The Forwells never had pop in their house, made their own sauces, and were "prepared to spend money" on food. As Bess said,

> We do spend money on things we like. And you have to do it early in your children's lives, or they're not going to eat it. So if you don't foster all of that, then you're going to be at the lowest common denominator, I think. And we like to think of ourselves

as not there, don't we? ... We'd like to be healthy and live forever
[laughs].

Nichole Hewey (fifty-one, African Canadian, working class) also noticed "the bad things" in other people's grocery carts: "If I see a cart
loaded with a bunch of junk, I just think to myself 'What are you eating?!'" Noreen Hardie (thirty-eight, white, upper middle class) signalled her own moral virtue by describing the objectionable contents
of children's school lunches: "Oh my God ... Kids would bring, like,
a little mini pop. I mean, it was just horrible ... Cinnamon rolls
and those Vachon cakes. I haven't even seen them for years!" Norah
Walters (thirty-five, white, working poor/impoverished) drew a symbolic boundary by describing herself as a "much better cook" than
her friends: "They're just not health conscious. They don't care how
much sugar goes in it or how much fat goes in it. They just slather it in
there and mix it up, and I'm thinking, 'Eww, gross.'"

Healthy eating discourses, then, can play a role in governing behaviour, and at the same time people can use them to demonstrate
their virtue and to distance themselves from others. Many participants
depicted themselves as closely following healthy eating standards,
but most also acknowledged that they fell short of their ideals. For
example, when asked how healthy their eating habits were, several
rated themselves at about eight out of ten. Others, however, acknowledged larger discrepancies. For some, this was accompanied by guilt
and self-blame. Norma Horne (forty-five, white, lower middle class),
who thought her eating habits were "fair to middle, not terrible, not
fantastic," was frustrated with her own lack of self-control:

> I get rebellious and just cook what I want to eat half the time ...
> I just get feeling tired and cranky, and I don't care about any
> of that [healthy, local, seasonal] stuff any more and I just want
> something that – you know, you're eating for psychological rea-
> sons instead of physical or political ones ... It's not supposed to
> be [that way]. You shouldn't make all your decisions like that.

Noni Webster (eighteen, white, lower middle class) was deeply embarrassed about revealing the inadequacy of her diet in a conversation
with us:

When you eat badly, you know it *[laughs]*. You just kind of hope nobody else realizes it. So when you're sitting down with somebody and they're asking you all these questions ... it really kind of takes you out in the open. It's like, oh damn! Not only does my family know, but this other person knows about this. This is terrible ... Another intelligent person looking at it and almost positively thinking to themselves, "That's not healthy!" Ugh, this is embarrassing!

Noni's comments evoke images of confession, which link food practices to modern techniques of self-discipline. As Foucault pointed out, confessing and self-monitoring act to discipline people and govern their behaviour (Foucault 1979, 1980; see also Coveney 2000).

Although some participants experienced shame and discontent when they didn't meet standards of healthy eating, this was not universal. A few happily acknowledged their lapses. Brady Forwell (fourteen, Euro-Canadian, lower middle class) and Bart Valverde (seventeen, white, upper middle class) said they did not eat very healthfully, with too few vegetables and too much fast food. Neither expressed concern about this. In addition, the Woods, especially the father, Nigel, were not concerned by their choices not to follow the healthy eating standards. In fact, he expressed resistance to it, stating that he would happily live a somewhat shorter time rather than have to be self-disciplined forever:

I don't want to be worried all the time and thinking, "Oh should I eat that?" Or only a spoonful of that. Or I must balance it with this thing I don't really feel like eating. 'Cause then meals won't become a joy any more. I love eating. I love food, I love the taste of it. I don't want it to be a time when it's a regimen that I must follow in order to be healthy. It would take all the joy out of eating, and it would take a lot of the joy out of an aspect of life I like. So if that costs me five years when I'm eighty, well –

Nigel and his wife, Nanette, seemed rather proud of their resistance to healthy eating "extremes," depicting food restriction as anti-pleasure.

In sum, social standards exhorting people to be responsible citizens and to follow healthy eating guidelines appeared to be countered primarily by the desire for pleasure. Whereas some participants, such as the Fagans, rejected the desire, others struck what they felt was an appropriate balance for their lives and context. Neither geographic location nor rural-urban differences affected this pattern. Further examination showed that gender and age were very salient in healthy eating discourses: adult women tended to be most engaged with healthy eating, and teenage boys (such as Brady Forwell and Bart Valverde) and men (such as Nigel Wood) were least engaged.

GENDER AND HEALTHY EATING DISCOURSES

In all four sites, healthy eating was predominantly – though not exclusively – understood as a feminine thing. The most explicit discussions of this occurred when participants sorted photos of foods into healthy and unhealthy categories, and into those more typically preferred by men or women. Regardless of location, age, or gender, most participants initially denied that foods were in any way gendered and then proceeded to sort the images into highly consistent categories of masculine (bacon cheeseburger, beef Wellington, pot roast, hot dog, pizza, and macaroni and cheese) or feminine (sushi, stir-fry, couscous, chicken soup, Korean food, fish, and spring green salad). Interestingly, the items perceived as masculine and feminine mapped almost perfectly onto those categorized as unhealthy and healthy, with the masculine foods typically seen as unhealthy (McPhail, Beagan, and Chapman 2012).

People in all sites explained that typically feminine foods were prettier, fancier, more "delicate," and especially lighter and healthier. Brooke Vessey (seventeen, white, upper middle class) noted that "women tend to try and eat a bit lighter more than men ... Instead of having a big hot dog, they'd have a salad. It's more of a womanly meal. Or the fish because they know that fish is really good for them." Similarly, Nelda Webster (fifty, white, lower middle class) said, "salad and soup, because it's light, girlie things." Light seemed to mean not only smaller portions, but also lower in fat and calories. As descriptors, "light" and "healthy" were used almost interchangeably.

Light, healthy eating emphasized vegetables. Reflecting on the foods she categorized as feminine, Bernadette Vickers (thirty-nine, Native and Irish Canadian, working poor/impoverished) connected light, healthy, feminine, and body weight. In sorting the photos, she remarked, "I've kind of categorized as more light food for the women. Like a stir-fry. This one looks like it has bean sprouts and lots of vegetables." Asked by the interviewer "When you say 'light' what do you mean?" she replied, "Probably more healthier, I guess. Because women are more concerned about their weight than men."

Brenda (forty-nine, Irish Canadian, working poor/impoverished) even more explicitly linked feminine foods with low weight: "We have a perception that vegetarian food is lower calories, less fat, healthier. It's going to keep you closer to your goal of being skinny." She suggested that women preferred lighter meals because, for them, "a criteria for being a successful person is that you're not fat." (Chapter 5 further explores how participants thought about diet, body image, and weight.)

When the women and girls talked about their *own* food practices, they echoed the gender patterns that equated health with thinness. They described eating "healthy" and "light" foods, primarily to reduce or maintain their weight. For example, Nuala Haldane (forty, white, working class) had adopted a healthy eating focus on produce and lean meats, "stuff that's good for you, that's not fattening." Similarly, Nalini Walters (nineteen, white, working poor/impoverished said that when she ate unhealthy foods, "It just puts weight on you." Concern with eating healthy low-calorie foods permeated almost all the interviews with female participants, regardless of their age, class, and location.

In contrast, typical masculine eating was depicted as unconcerned with health or weight. Almost everyone described men as reluctant to eat vegetables, the agreed-upon cornerstone of both healthy eating and maintaining weight control. Masculine diets were characterized as meat-centred, hearty, heavy, and filling. As Brenda Voisey stated, "Men like heavier food. I think men like more meat-and-potatoes food ... a heartier meal." Regardless of age or gender, almost everyone associated men and meat, especially beef. Classifying meat as masculine and vegetables as feminine was occasionally rationalized on the basis of men's physical labour, even though this was acknowledged as often inaccurate: "I think men in our culture have been brought up by mothers who say, 'You need hearty food' ... You work hard and you eat hard kind of thing" (Beryl Fredericks, thirty-eight, white, lower middle class).

Just as the women echoed stereotyped associations of femininity and light eating in describing their own eating patterns, the men and boys were also depicted as meat-eaters. Bernice Valverde (forty-three, white, upper middle class) acknowledged the link between meat consumption and masculinity but was exasperated with the amount of meat that her son and male partner ate: "There's too much meat in the household right now!" The family had been vegetarian for many years, until her son Bart became a teenager and "his body just needed something else." Seventeen-year-old Bart reported, "I started eating meat, and he [father] was just, like, 'Yes!' He started eating a little more."

Participant associations among masculinity, meat, and the dismissal of healthy eating are supported by studies that suggest the rejection of healthy eating is virtually a defining characteristic of masculinity (Gough and Conner 2006; Mróz et al. 2011a, 2011b) and that engaging in healthy eating, especially for weight loss, can threaten a man's portrayal of masculinity (Lyons 2009). It is often socially unacceptable for men to admit concern with body image (Gough 2007; Monaghan 2008) or an aversion to meat (Sobal 2005). Frequently, men who diet for health or weight loss insist that their female partners are "in charge" of food preparation and nutrition, maintaining the notion that dieting is feminine (de Souza and Ciclitira 2005; Mróz et al. 2011a).

It is important to note that four of the ten adult men whom we interviewed in British Columbia and Nova Scotia were focused on consuming "healthy" and "light" foods. For three of them, this was the result of health scares such as a stroke or diabetes. Niall Haggerty (forty-five, white, lower middle class) struggled to lower his consumption of sugar and fat after a diabetes diagnosis. Only one adult man, Burt Fitzgerald, discussed food restriction and healthy eating solely in terms of weight loss. Fitzgerald (forty-three, white, upper middle class) and his wife followed the "Body for Life" plan, emphasizing salad and white (as opposed to red) meat consumption: "I'll have salad with maybe some tuna, canned tuna, or salad with maybe sliced meat like ham or chicken breast, with a little bit of dressing." It is noteworthy that Burt was upper middle class – other research indicates that men can afford to compromise their displays of masculinity in some ways when their social status is assured in other ways (Connell and Messerschmidt 2005; Sellaeg and Chapman 2008). In general, adult male interviewees did not talk much about healthy eating, though Nigel Wood did display active resistance to it, as mentioned above.

Most of the twenty-one boys whom we interviewed in British Columbia and Nova Scotia thought that their eating practices were reasonable but felt that they "could eat more vegetables" (Naish White, sixteen, Acadian Canadian, working class). Bernard Valeriani (thirteen, Italian and Native, working poor/impoverished) contrasted his own healthy eating with the diets of his friends: "Girls eat healthier than boys, usually. I like spring green salad, but I have a lot of friends and they don't really like salad that much." Other boys thought they ate fairly healthfully, particularly at home, and emphasized that they tried to avoid "junk food." Only one, Bart Valverde, explicitly dismissed healthy eating, commenting that the healthier you get, "the more you jeopardize deliciousness." Barrett Vale (sixteen, El Salvadoran Canadian, lower middle class) captured the emphasis on masculine meat eating and its associated lack of investment in healthy eating:

> I love my protein, my meats, because I'm very carnivorous, but I still try to get all of my fruits and vegetables and stuff like that. Unfortunately, if it comes down just to a snack, I'll probably have, like, cereal over a pear or an apple or whatever. So I try to eat healthy, but, you know, I'm human and I like to indulge every once in a while. Or a lot *[laughs]*.

These patterns held true among boys regardless of geographic location.

In sum, the interviews suggest that healthy eating is generally perceived as a feminine concern, mostly because of its association with weight control. Standards of masculinity that promote large, heavy, meat-centred meals may set men up for increased health risks. However, there is also evidence that some men and boys *do* engage with healthy eating practices, particularly if they have experienced health problems. Nonetheless, the key point here is that because femininity is strongly associated with healthy eating, women and girls can more readily present themselves as both "good citizens" and "good women/ girls," whereas for men and boys enacting "good citizen" through healthy eating contradicts their gender performance of masculinity.

A GENDERED DISCOURSE: BEING A "GOOD MOTHER"

For women, social expectations regarding healthy eating extend beyond taking responsibility for their own health to taking care of their families. Most adult women participants constituted themselves as "good mothers" through providing healthy food for their families and actively encouraging them to eat healthfully. Nuala Haldane, for example, said that even when she was short of money, "I'm still going to give my kids fresh fruit and fresh vegetables and stuff that's healthy for them. I'm going to try my best anyways with what I've got." Norma Horne (forty-five, white, lower middle class) made "more of an effort" to buy organic produce for her daughter than she did for herself.

Beryl Fredericks cited the gendered aspects of concern for healthy eating:

> I'm always trying to get most of the men in my immediate family to eat more vegetables. You know, recently I said to Blaine [her son], "You are fifteen. You need more salad on your plate than that small amount that was good enough when you were ten" ... We [women] are the ones that worry more about what everyone is eating.

Some women acted as "gatekeepers," bringing only (or mostly) healthy food into the home and ensuring that it was always available. Belva Vernon (fifty, white New Zealand Canadian, upper middle class) tried to make her house "a bit of an oasis of healthy foods," arguing, "if there are foods that are problems for you, don't have them around the house." Getting everyone to eat healthfully involved work – adding certain ingredients to recipes or preparing disliked healthy foods in ways the family would accept.

Most participants took for granted maternal roles in promoting healthy eating, but it was also understood as a *responsibility* of mothering. Bronwyn Vale (forty-one, white, lower middle class) knew that she could not control what her son ate outside the home, "So that makes me feel even more responsible for being really healthy at home ... I feel like I need to be sure they get their vitamins when they're here." Beryl Fredericks had felt absolutely responsible for her children's health in the past. When they became ill, she asked herself "What did I do wrong?" She felt that she had "failed in this little way" when she bought packaged cookies or other foods with "questionable ingredients" for her children: "I've spent agonizing amounts of time in the past stressing about everything that my kids are putting into their mouths and spending five or six hours a day cooking. You know, from the raw foods and spending so much money on cold-pressed safflower oil and things like that." At the time of her interviews, Beryl had relinquished some of that responsibility, trying to feel "satisfied by the act of providing what I see is a pretty healthy diet."

Like Beryl, most women in all four sites thought that indulging in the occasional unhealthy food was acceptable, as long as their children's diets were *mostly* healthy. Sometimes unhealthy foods were convenient or a treat. At other times, they were a way to get a child to eat *something*. As Beatrice Valeriani said, "I try to limit [my son's] pop and limit his sugars, but sometimes with the working and lack of time it's easier to just buy a pizza, and you know he's going to eat it, right?" But because encouraging healthy eating enabled women to constitute themselves as good mothers, most felt virtuous when they provided healthy food for their families. Natalia Warshawski (forty-seven, white, lower middle class) talked about making smoothies for her children: "I feel good about it because I know the kids are getting their milk, their fruit serving. It's just very healthful."

Interviews with teenagers also provided extensive evidence of mothers' roles in supporting healthy eating, including numerous comments about Mom as the provider of healthy food and the main source of nutrition knowledge. In explaining why her family always had salad at dinner, Brooke Vessey (seventeen, white, upper middle class) commented that "Mom's like that" and added,

> My mom is very conscious about what we eat and what and when
> we should eat it ... I've been brought up that way to sort of think
> consciously about what I eat ... My mom's always been conscious
> of our weight, and she wants me to be healthy, and my dad, so I
> think she's just looking out for herself and her family.

Brooke's mention of her father, like Beryl Frederick's comment about her attempts to influence the men in her family, suggests that though women focused mainly on their children, adult men were sometimes included among those who needed care, seen as otherwise uninterested in healthy eating. Brooke Vessey reinforced this idea in stating that "me and my dad like to indulge in other things when my mom's not around." In a few families, such as the Fagans, healthy eating was jointly enforced by both parents. Only in the Wood family did the father seem to encourage it more than the mother.

In dominant social standards, mothering includes responsibility for family food habits, training family members in healthy eating, and producing a healthy family (Ristovski-Slijepcevic, Chapman, and Beagan 2010). Regardless of social or geographic location, many mothers had internalized expectations that they monitor both their own food practices and those of their children and male partners; this entailed controlling the foods that came into the house, providing healthy role models, and acting as nutrition educators. Their behaviour exemplifies governmentality as described by Foucault, where people take on responsibility for regulating their own actions, monitoring and encouraging others to act in accountable ways and producing themselves as moral, ethical, or good citizens (in this case, good mothers who are properly gendered) (Lupton 1996; Coveney 1998, 2000; Ristovski-Slijepcevic, Chapman, and Beagan 2010). Mothers who felt they were not living up to these standards often felt guilty or inadequate.

LIFE STAGE: TEENS AND HEALTHY EATING

Just as healthy eating is seen as a concern of women and mothers, and resistance to it is depicted as inherently masculine, the life stages of childhood and adolescence are understood as entailing little interest in healthy eating (Taylor, Evers, and McKenna 2005). When participants sorted photos into "adult" and "teen" foods, there was strong consensus that the bacon cheeseburger, macaroni and cheese, tacos, hot dog, grilled cheese sandwich, and pizza were typically teen foods. Baljit Virk (seventeen, South Asian Canadian, working class) explained that they were all "unhealthy foods that teenagers mostly eat." Seventeen-year-old Brooke Vessey noted, "I think when you're young, you're, like, 'Oh I'm young, I can eat whatever I want. I'm not going to gain weight. I'm young and, like, nothing's going to happen.'" Participants emphasized that in addition to being unconcerned about health, teens *like* convenient and tasty foods: "It's easier, it's tastier, it's badder for you" (Nailah Warshawski, sixteen, white, lower middle class).

For some teens, indifference to healthy eating was also apparent when they talked about their *own* habits, either because they never mentioned health and nutrition or because they specifically said they did not care about healthy eating. Bart Valverde (seventeen, white, upper middle class), for example, did not take health into account when he made food choices, as long as food "tastes good and is not complete junk food." Similarly, Neha Hewey (eighteen, white and African Canadian, working class) said nonchalantly, "We never eat healthy at all ... It never worries me and that's why I'm getting fat now ... I don't really pay attention to what I eat."

But overall, in all four sites teens' responses to healthy eating discourses were more complex than simple rejection or inattention. Some distinguished themselves as healthy eaters, drawing a symbolic boundary in opposition to the discourse that teens do not care about healthy eating, claiming – sometimes matter-of-factly and sometimes proudly – that they generally ate a healthy diet. Baljit Virk, for instance, who said that teenagers mostly opted for unhealthy food, described his own habits as "very healthy. I never eat out. I never buy junk food." Similarly, Newlyn Henderson (thirteen, white, upper middle class) stated, "I think I eat healthier than most. There's never any really unhealthy food in the house. There's always a healthy option. There's no chips and high-fat food. And we don't eat deep-fried food and we don't go out very often. And we always have fruit and vegetables and stuff."

Interestingly, the teenagers in the Walters family were actively pressuring their mother, Norah (thirty-five, white, working poor/ impoverished), to adopt healthier choices. When their school adopted healthy eating policies and they started asking her for healthy foods, she changed her approach: "I said, 'Fine, if you want to eat that way, we'll go shopping,' and I just let them pick what they thought was healthy. And surprisingly, they did a really, really great job ... I was the one that had the biggest adjustment."

More frequently, though, teens presented inconsistent messages about healthy eating. They talked about times or ways in which they ate healthfully, appearing to feel good about themselves for doing so, but somewhat ruefully acknowledged other times when they ate easy or tempting foods. Nailah Warshawski (sixteen, white, lower middle class) described a typical day's eating as "generally pretty healthy; we don't eat a lot of crap. Crap meaning unhealthy food." But she also said she "would like to eat slightly healthier. More fruits and vegetables, because I don't get enough, I don't think." She noted, "Sometimes it's easy to grab something crappy or something unhealthy, and so that's just what we do." Noni Webster (eighteen, white, lower middle class) said that her eating habits were typically poor – not a lot of vegetables and fruits – but was happy to tell the interviewer that she was currently eating well: "For about a week or so, I've just been really on the good track. Like I just, one day I woke up and was like, 'Yeah, I'm just going to eat right now' ... I've just been going crazy with the salads."

She expected that her new eating style would last as long as it tasted good because "it's a lot about taste for me. If I can keep the taste there, it's no problem." Nolan Howell (eighteen, white, working poor/impoverished) also prioritized taste over health but tried to eat one healthy meal a day to compensate for his other unhealthy habits – eating "a lot of crap" and not exercising. Saying that he ate apples, oranges, and spinach "once in a while," he added, "I balance it out with a heavy diet of grease and saturated fats, MSG." When asked if he wanted to change this, he spoke candidly and reflexively about the long-term impact of his diet: "I want to because I know that in here [pointing to his chest], the plaque's building up. But the thing is I don't see myself gaining much weight or becoming unable to run around. So it's harder for me to tell myself that it's killing me slowly. But I know it is."

Brooke Vessey generally presented herself as a healthy eater, which she attributed to her mother's efforts. However, she admitted that she sometimes chose unhealthy foods and said that she needed to monitor her eating practices, even though this was difficult to do consistently. As she put it, watching her food intake was "always in the back of my mind when I'm eating, [but] sometimes I don't listen to what I'm thinking."

Given the qualitative nature of our study, it was impossible to determine which demographic characteristics would predict which teens generally ignored or resisted healthy eating messages and which tended to embrace them. There were no clear patterns by geographic location and no rural-urban differences. However, we did note some trends

(McPhail, Chapman, and Beagan 2011; Johnston, Rodney, and Szabo 2012), especially with regard to gender. Pressures to eat healthfully appeared to be felt most strongly by the young women, particularly when linked with maintaining a slim body. Brooke Vessey explained, "I think guys aren't as conscious of healthy eating. It's just there's not as much pressure to be, like, fit and thin and everything." Some parents also identified the ways in which teen culture could encourage positive eating behaviours. Bette Falcon (thirty-three, Cree and French Canadian, lower middle class) thought that gendered peer pressure encouraged her sixteen-year-old daughter Blaise to eat healthy food, which was seen as "cool" among her friends. While at home Blaise would eat an entire pizza, but with her friends she ordered "salads or Thai stir-fry." Bette commented,

> They try to be really "healthy" ... They don't want to be perceived as eating this junk food where people are, "You're going to get fat if you eat that." Or teased or stuff like that. So, the girls, when they are with the guys, when they are together, Blaise might have a small portion of food. Then she'll wait till they're gone and ... then she gets into the comfort foods.

Bette connected this peer pressure to social messages concerning slenderness. However, the relationship between gender and body image is more complex than this, as will be examined in Chapter 5.

CONCLUSION

This chapter reveals various responses to the dominant discourse of healthy eating. Every participant was familiar with it, and most reiterated its main points. Some subscribed to alternative or traditional discourses, and some resisted healthy eating, usually from the stance of food-as-pleasure.

Nonetheless, the discourse was so pervasive that individuals could employ it to convey their social identities. Adhering to it enabled them to see themselves as moral people, whereas deviating from it could prompt self-criticism. Some who resisted it proudly portrayed themselves as defiant and ungovernable.

Gender and age played a role as well. Healthy, "light" eating was regarded as inherently feminine, a fact that permitted women and girls to solidify their feminine social identities. For men and boys, however, healthy eating could undermine masculinity. Mothers were expected to assume responsibility for the healthful eating of everyone in the family. Here, too, they could construct themselves – and be constructed by others – as good or bad mothers, depending on how they fed their families. To some extent, teens were expected to disregard healthy eating, but they did not consistently report doing so.

Ultimately, the healthy eating discourse was central to how the participants thought about and portrayed themselves in the social world. Eating is not just about personal preference, and everyone is required to negotiate the discourse. This is not to say that it dictates our actions – as we have seen, adherence is rarely perfect, and creative engagement certainly occurs. Rather, alternative discourses, including those of masculinity and adolescence, provide some people with more or less freedom to engage with and counter the healthy eating discourse. And, of course, anyone can refuse to follow the rules, though this risks being cast as bad, as less virtuous, or as failing to meet social standards.

2

eating ethically

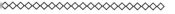

The Keefe Family

THE KEEFES ARE a white, high-income (over $150,000 annually), upper-middle-class family who live in a gentrified area of Kingston, Ontario. Kent Keefe (forty-five) is a family physician; his wife, Kara (forty-five), is an artist and art teacher. The family's diet revolves around the belief that local and organic foods are good for the health of individuals and the earth. All the Keefes embrace the politics of local eating and prefer homemade, non-processed foods. Kara, who does all the shopping for the family, purchases primarily organic meat, dairy, and produce from local farmers. Income allows this family to prioritize its political and ethical beliefs. As Kara puts it, "I don't spend as little money as I can. But I guess for me, and us, food is a priority. It's worth it for me, to spend money on food."

Kara also wants to impress upon her children the importance of eating locally grown and organic food. She seeks "to give the kids a sense of where

. . . .

This chapter was co-authored with Alexandra Rodney and Michelle Szabo.

their food comes from, and knowing the people that actually produce food." Aged fifteen and thirteen, Karl and Kylie are both articulate about the politics and ethics of eating. Karl in particular is vehement about not eating processed foods (which he calls "processed crap") and was a vegetarian until shortly before our interviews. In response to his preferences, as well as her own aversion to meat, Kara serves very little of it for family meals.

The Keefes believe that they eat differently from other families. Kara spoke about being "horrified" by the lunches that her children's friends brought to school and added that her children are sometimes regarded as "freaks" because their lunches contain no processed food. Kylie was "shocked" by friends who brought Lunchables and pop to school, and the fact that their families rarely ate together. In contrast, the Keefes put considerable emphasis on connecting with each other through food, displaying much pride and respect for each other's food choices. The teens express their appreciation for eating meals together, and for Kara's cooking, with Karl noting that "everything is made from scratch, which I love."

The Keefes also emphasize the importance of connecting to local food systems, through visiting farmers' markets and participating in the local food movement. Although Kylie is only thirteen, she is very knowledgeable about local food. She notes that it is readily available because of Kingston's proximity to agricultural land. She also links income levels, eating habits, and food options, suggesting that "levels of wealth translate to what the people eat. I guess the bigger the city, the more dynamic the food is." In essence, the Keefes' awareness of political and moral issues leads them to prioritize particular ethics in their shopping, cooking, and eating. They attempt to buy locally and organically, attend to animal welfare issues, connect to producers, and consume homemade, non-processed food.

· · · *The Radanovic Family*

THE RADANOVICS, A low-income ($22,000 annually), Serbian Canadian family of two, live in a housing co-operative in Toronto's North Riverdale neighbourhood. Tatjana (fifty-three) is a landscape architect, and her son, Teodor (seventeen), is in his final year of high school. The family immigrated to Canada from Serbia when he was four. Tatjana is committed to eating organic, local, and unprocessed foods. However, given her limited income, maintaining this stance has required creativity.

Tatjana has a passion for growing food, which infuses her work, recreation, family life, and volunteer efforts. She is committed to community involvement and raising consciousness about links between the health of people and the planet. She believes that everyone should have access to local and organic food, and that communities are morally obligated to take care of all citizens' food needs: "I've thought a lot about food and I really believe that food is a big part of our life, and I think we should pay more attention ... to be connected in some different way and taking time for foods." Tatjana majored in horticulture at university and now works with non-profit organizations, developing community and rooftop gardens. She volunteers extensively at community gardens and grows additional food in her garden at home. As a result, she produces much of her food herself and is also given food grown by friends and colleagues.

Three years ago, Tatjana was diagnosed with ovarian cancer. After a hysterectomy, she opted to focus on food to support her recovery, instead of chemotherapy or radiation: "Since I am an environmentalist and don't trust chemicals at all, that is not the path for me. You have to trust your medicine ... So I chose herbalism, I chose homeopathy, and food, and change of lifestyle." She was on a raw food diet for eight months, eating only food grown by herself or her friends.

Tatjana tries to be self-sustaining and cooks mostly from scratch. She would like to shop exclusively at organic grocery stores for items that she can't grow, but her low income prevents this. Employing a cheaper alternative, she barters with friends for some products or buys food in bulk at low-end grocery stores. When Teodor was younger, she cooked for another family with two working parents; in exchange, they purchased the food, which both families shared every evening.

Teodor's eating habits evoke some tension in the house. In sharp contrast to Tatjana, he prefers convenience food, especially with his friends, and has little interest in gardening: "I don't really eat many vegetables and fruits. More of a junk food guy ... It's just convenient. And I know I like the junk food." What the two do share, however, is a love for Serbian dishes. Tatjana attributes her interest in eating whole, fresh foods and sharing food with others to her Serbian heritage.

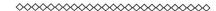

THE CASE STUDIES of the Keefe and Radanovic families illustrate concerns about local and organic food, gardening, and connecting to others through food – issues that are part of a larger social discourse of "ethical" eating (Beagan, Ristovski-Slijepcevic, and Chapman 2010; Morgan 2010; Johnston, Szabo, and Rodney 2011; Biltekoff 2013). This is not always completely distinct from healthy eating. Organic food, for example, can be part of healthy eating but can also be an ethical concern, linking food to care for the planet and all who live on it.

THEORETICAL FRAMING

Thinking about ethical eating* as a socially constructed discourse helps us appreciate how systems of thought organize our ideas of eating and shape which food issues appear most pressing in the public sphere (Johnston and Baumann 2010; Biltekoff 2013). The contemporary ethical eating discourse is characterized not by a universal sense of right and wrong in relation to food choices, but by the selective prominence of certain issues – such as organic certification, local provenance, and the humane treatment of animals in food production (as for free-run eggs). Concerns that might also be deemed ethical do not figure as prominently in the North American discourse, where environmental issues tend to overshadow those of hunger, food security, and the exploitation of agricultural labour (Johnston and Baumann 2010). The pre-eminence of environmental issues demonstrates that the ethical eating discourse (like all discourses) contains numerous contradictions (Sassatelli 2006; Johnston 2008). For example, green campaigns to "eat local" can operate at cross-purposes with social justice campaigns to support fair-trade farming (Morgan 2010). In addition, privileged perspectives tend to be normalized and presented as classless – despite the structural inequalities that make it difficult for marginalized groups to eat with maximum efficiency, healthfulness, deliciousness, and distinction (Johnston and Baumann 2010; Biltekoff 2013).

. . . .

* To be clear, our objective in this chapter is not to judge which food consumption practices are inherently ethical or unethical. Our goal is to study how they are shaped by the broad discourse of ethical eating and how participants articulated and creatively engaged with it. For reasons of readability, we don't enclose the term "ethical" in quotation marks, but readers should remember that the practices of the ethical consumption discourse are not inherently more ethical than others.

We employed the concept of the cultural repertoire to better understand the ethical eating discourse (Swidler 1986, 2001; Lamont 1992; Tilly 1993). This concept enabled us to avoid viewing the discourse as a monolithic force or "given object" (Adams and Raisborough 2010, 259) and to appreciate how actors employed its components in everyday life. In this chapter, we refer to an "ethical eating repertoire" that involves a broad set of culinary practices, ideas, and habits. Indeed, ethical eating is neither singular nor static – it is multi-faceted, dynamic, and discursive. In our interviews, we sought to determine which elements of an ethical eating repertoire were most salient in participants' lives, which were relatively minor, and which factors shaped engagement.

The elements of an ethical eating repertoire are not universally held; they differ geographically (Sassatelli and Davolio 2010; Bondy and Talwar 2011) and are constantly evolving, and thus our findings reveal consumption practices in a particular place and time. Focusing on interviewees in Ontario, we explore how social class and ethnicity, as well as geographic location and local food culture, affected people's involvement with ethical eating. We attend to how geographic place – where people lived, shopped, and ate – influenced their engagement with the repertoire. The presence of stores that sold ethical products, and residents' awareness of them, is related to ethical food purchases (Popkin, Duffey, and Gordon-Larsen 2005; Brown, Dury, and Holdsworth 2009; Beagan, Ristovski-Slijepcevic, and Chapman 2010). Such businesses tend to cluster in more affluent neighbourhoods, impeding access for non-residents or users of public transportation (Ellaway and Macintyre 2000; Moore and Diez Roux 2006; Baker, Hamshaw, and Kolodinsky 2009). For low-income people, access, distance, and cost hinder engagement with ethical eating (Smith and Morton 2009). At the same time, ethical eating repertoires are shaped by the cultures of food and consumption, which can exist geographically at various scales (neighbourhood, region, nation) (DeSoucey 2010; Oluwabamide and Akpan 2010). For example, there is some evidence that a culture of ethical eating may be stronger on Canada's West Coast than the East Coast, in turn leading to greater prevalence of ethical stores and markets (Beagan, Ristovski-Slijepcevic, and Chapman 2010).

In addition, an emerging body of literature suggests that ethical consumption is a highly gendered practice (see, for example, Little,

Ilbery, and Watts 2009; Cairns, Johnston, and MacKendrick 2013). It connects strongly to the notion of good mothering, which was introduced in the previous chapter. Not only do women perform most of the foodwork in Canadian families (Beagan et al. 2008), but they also appear to be held (and hold themselves) primarily responsible for ensuring their ethical consumption (Cairns, Johnston, and MacKendrick 2013). Note that both Kara Keefe and Tatjana Radanovic emphasized their desire to serve ethically produced foods and to instill the same values in their children. The ability to engage in this version of good mothering, however, is strongly influenced by social position, especially income and class.

PARTICIPANTS, PLACES, AND APPROACH TO ANALYSIS

We did not endeavour to recruit families who were specifically engaged with ethical eating, but we noted degrees and types of involvement as we analyzed the interview transcripts. The four Ontario communities that are the focus of this chapter are the Toronto neighbourhoods of South Parkdale and North Riverdale, Kingston, and Prince Edward County. South Parkdale is a gentrifying working-class neighbourhood that is ethnically and racially diverse. Our ten South Parkdale families had a range of incomes and ethnic backgrounds. North Riverdale, a more affluent, middle- or upper-middle-class community, is predominantly white. Its retail area includes a green-living store, farmers' markets, and a large grocery store (the Big Carrot) that sells organic, local, and "natural" food. The ten families in this neighbourhood had a range of incomes, and most were white.

Kingston is a mid-sized city with a relatively well-educated population but a major split in income levels, with significant numbers of very high-income and very low-income households. Its population is predominantly white. Kingston hosts one of the most vibrant downtown areas in Ontario, with numerous restaurants, specialty food shops, and a well-established farmers' market. Our thirteen Kingston families had a range of incomes and ethnic backgrounds. Prince Edward County, which is rural and primarily agricultural, lies about half an hour west of Kingston. Typical of the area, the nine families from "the County" were low to middle income, and all identified as white of European heritage. Overall, the Ontario families were quite diverse. Eleven were high-income earners, twenty-three were low income, and eight were in between.

Beginning our interview analysis by looking at the ways in which participants discussed ethical eating, we discovered that many had obviously drawn from a common repertoire with recognizable themes. Johnston and Baumann (2010, 138–63) argue that the major North American themes in this repertoire are local provenance and seasonality, organics, sustainability, and animal welfare. Minor themes are social justice, labour issues, and community development. All were present in our data. We then considered how participants' comments were related to the dominant discourse of ethical eating and also noted instances in which they spoke about other, less pervasive moral concerns that influenced their food practices.

We categorized interview transcripts according to the relative presence/absence of the prevailing ethical consumption themes. In keeping with the concept of a cultural repertoire, we made note of interviewee food practices (routines, habits) as well as their ideas, knowledge, and awareness of the food system more generally. We defined knowledge of ethical eating as a general awareness of its key ideas, debates, and aspirations (such as understanding that eating locally is thought to reduce carbon emissions). Practices included the fundamental activities of the repertoire (such as buying local food or avoiding heavily packaged food).

Families were categorized as having weak, moderate, or strong engagement with the repertoire. Weak engagement was indicated by its very minimal presence in the interviews, either as knowledge or practice. Moderately engaged families drew on some key themes of ethical eating but with a certain tension – perhaps only a few were mentioned, or significant knowledge was accompanied by minimal practice. Strongly engaged families displayed substantial knowledge and practices. In general, our interview data revealed that involvement was broadly dispersed. Of the forty-two families discussed in this chapter, twenty-two were weakly, nine moderately, and eleven strongly engaged (such as the Keefes). It is worth briefly noting that most of the strongly engaged families were upper middle class (seven) and that most of their moderately engaged counterparts were lower middle class (five). Most weakly engaged families were working class or working poor (thirteen).

To be clear, we are classifying engagement with just one version of ethical eating. There are many ways of expressing ethics through food practices, and the dominant ethical eating repertoire is neither unique nor superior. It simply enjoys ascendancy.

THE DOMINANT ETHICAL EATING REPERTOIRE

Three themes characterized the dominant ethical eating discourse: eco-eating, restricting meat, and community relations. These figured strongly among "highly engaged" interviewees. Like other work on ethical consumption (such as Johnston and Baumann 2010, 160), our interviews revealed that environmental considerations, or "green" issues, were a major aspect of the ethical eating repertoire. Many participants primarily conceptualized ethical eating as involving local and/or organic foods, and frequently equated it with healthy eating. They connected certain food choices with environmental damage, such as carbon emissions from food transport and the harmful effects of pesticides and factory farming. The Keefes, introduced above, exemplify consumers for whom organic and local considerations influenced shopping and eating habits. Their diet was grounded in the belief that local and organic foods are good for both people and the planet. As Kara Keefe, age thirteen, explained, "the closer food is to the earth, and the shorter time it's taken to get to you, the better it is." Many other participants thought similarly about ethical food purchasing, such as Tristan Rousseau (seventeen, white, upper middle class). In describing his family's habits, he said, "We try to stay organic whenever we can and local definitely for fruits and stuff. We try to stay with what's in season and what's from Canada, from Ontario ... Organic, less pesticide and stuff on it, and local stuff's usually more fresh and environmentally hasn't been brought that far. So, less fuel spent on one peach."

As Tristan made clear, organic and local food consumption were linked to environmental sustainability. Another key part of the ethical eating repertoire involved understanding and engaging with the tension between organic foods (grown without chemical pesticides, herbicides, and fertilizers) and locally produced foods (which travel a shorter distance from field to plate). Ted Rodger (fifty-two, white, upper middle class) voiced his awareness of this issue and of the imperatives of the hundred-mile diet: "I'll buy organic. I'll buy local over

California organics, and I try to keep things that are close to that one-hundred-mile radius. I try to buy local as much as I can. And if I can't, I will buy organic, but I try to buy Canadian produce."

Limiting meat consumption was another significant part of the ethical eating repertoire. Several participants had been vegetarians in the past, some were currently vegetarians, and some made a point of eating little meat. Although interviewees spoke about restricting meat for health reasons, they also discussed the effects of the meat industry on the environment and criticized factory farming and animal mistreatment more generally. Therese Parsons (forty-five, white, upper middle class) touched on all these themes when explaining why she limited meat consumption and bought organic or free-range meat:

> I think all the reasons that people have for not eating meat or preferring free range as opposed to factory, I think they are all valid … If I think about the animal welfare, I'm like, yeah, that's terrible. Or if I think about the manner in which they are processed … I think this [free-range and/or organic meat] is much [better]. And from an environmental point of view, probably especially for bigger animals like cows and stuff, that [view] would be the one I would put the most importance on … you know, smaller farms, better life for the animals. They're better looked after, the quality [of the meat] is going to be better.

In some instances, the reasons for choosing vegetarianism changed over time, revealing an overlap between health and specific ethical issues. Karine Clements (fifty-one, white, lower middle class) said that her vegetarianism "started with social justice, then went to health as it helped with my gallbladder problem, then went to a concern with organics and ethical eating." Tandy Price (forty-nine, European and Middle Eastern, lower middle class), who was strongly engaged with ethical eating, connected her reduced meat consumption to global hunger: "I'm trying to do my part … I read somewhere … that if we reduced our meat consumption by 10 percent, we'd have enough grain left over to feed every hungry person in the world. And 10 percent isn't much." This type of concern was rare in our sample, mentioned by only one other participant, Tracey Raikatuji (fifteen, Japanese Canadian, lower middle class). Her vegetarianism was prompted by unease about factory farming and the belief that "the amount of grain that goes to feed the cows could feed the entire world population."

A less prominent element of the repertoire focused on enhancing social connections and building community. Social issues were mentioned much less frequently than environmental motivations and were most commonly framed through a local lens rather than linked to global inequality, poverty, or food insecurity. For example, some participants wanted to support businesses and economic development in their communities, which was usually articulated through support for farmers' markets. Twenty-four of the forty-two families mentioned visiting farmers' markets, and higher-class participants did so with greater regularity, although it is important to mention that some lower-class interviewees would have shopped at markets if they could afford it.

Interviewees also showed concern about community building through their preference for small, local businesses rather than large supermarkets. Many families discussed the importance of knowing who grew or processed their food. For Kingston-area families (such as the Keefes) who felt relatively connected to rural growers, this took the form of knowing local farmers. Keira Karsten (thirty-two, white, working class) spoke about how her shopping experience was improved by purchasing food at Prince Edward County farmers' markets: "It's interaction with people and with the actual farmers, and since we love Prince Edward County, it has a place in our hearts. The farmers are more involved. The farmers help you pick things out and try things before you purchase them as a family, which is really nice. At the grocery store, you can't just go around sampling everything."

For urban residents, connecting with food producers often meant building relationships with small neighbourhood retailers. Tawna Parsons (twelve, white, upper middle class) mentioned the importance of her father's connection with their local butcher: "We have this one butcher and my dad knows him really well ... [He] gets free bones from this guy." Her mother, Therese, spoke in more detail about the value of such links: "I think this is much more fun shopping than the supermarket. And, you know, you talk to the people who make the stuff or grow it and bring it ... I like knowing the people. You know, I think there's something about that that's worthwhile." Other participants mentioned wanting to "keep the money in the [local] economy," feeling greatest trust in local business people, and being able to find out more details about products than in a supermarket.

Concern about fair wages and working conditions, both domestically and abroad, was a minor element of the ethical consumption repertoire, but a few participants did discuss it. Tandy Price, who was strongly engaged with ethical eating, described her reasons for patronizing local businesses:

> I'd rather support a small-business person who's trying to keep their family together than some corporation that's making billions ... And I just know that workers, say, in Mexico aren't being paid as good a wage ... I paid more for tomatoes coming from Ontario than I did for Mexican tomatoes, and I didn't mind, I just didn't buy as many as I might have bought.

ETHICAL EATING: PRIVILEGE AND PLACE

Participants who were highly engaged in the dominant mode of ethical eating were all middle class (mainly upper middle but also lower middle) and predominantly white.* In families with high incomes and high education, interviewees were familiar with the socio-cultural/political/philosophical ideas behind ethical eating and significantly incorporated them into their food practices. Like the Keefe family, the Parsonses, upper-middle-class Torontonians, bought mostly local, organic, and free-range products. They were concerned with health and with the environmental and animal welfare issues related to factory farming (such as over-fishing and water contamination from factory farm run-off). They enjoyed buying seasonally from farmers' markets and prioritized getting to know local food store owners. At only twelve years old, Tawna Parsons was impressively knowledgeable about ethical eating, speaking in detail about topics such as feeding corn to cows, who were "supposed to eat grass." Both mother and daughter spoke with pride and enthusiasm about the family's cooking and shopping habits; Therese's eyes lit up when she described being

. . . .

* Only two highly engaged families were not white; one was of South Asian descent, and the other described itself as of mixed white, Middle Eastern, and African heritage.

"inspired" to cook by the "lovely" shapes and colours of foods at a favourite farmers' market.

Similarly, in Prince Edward County, the Chirnian family was concerned with ethical eating on a philosophical and practical level. Though divorce had reduced their income, Kristal Chirnian (forty-two, white, upper middle class) and her children were strongly motivated to eat organic, local, and unprocessed foods, which they understood as closely associated with healthy eating. They felt that local food and local eating connected them to the County. Kristal said, "I have a sense of food from Prince Edward County being food from home. I live in the County; it feels good to eat in the County." The Chirnians had moved from Toronto, where they had learned to appreciate food variety and ethics/politics, including vegetarianism and veganism. Daughter Kallie (fifteen) and son Kamer (thirteen) enjoyed fresh produce from the County in the summertime and felt attuned to seasonality.

In contrast to families such as the Parsonses and the Chirnians, the working poor were unlikely to engage with the dominant ethical consumption repertoire. In fact, all had low involvement with it. Class and income played a role here, as ethical food products are expensive. Some interviewees who were interested in buying organic and local did not do so because of the cost. Tatjana Radanovic noted, "I love going to farmers' markets and shopping, but that is the most expensive way to buy things." Trudy Patterson (sixty, white, working poor/impoverished) said of farmers' markets, "Sometimes I think they're charging much more" and termed their prices unreasonable "for your everyday person." Kennedy Clements (thirteen, white, lower middle class) had a similar impression: "When you see poorer people and the food they're eating, it's usually the cheaper stuff. You have to have money to get the kind of food that's really good food. Organic food is really expensive."

Although many families had relatively high incomes, only one upper-middle-class family talked about purchasing organic meat and dairy exclusively. This is not to say that price and income were all-determining. Some high-income families rejected ethical eating. Thelma Read (forty-seven, white, upper middle class) wasn't willing to pay a premium for organics, because she and her husband thought they might just be "BS." Conversely, some lower-income participants evolved strategies for eating ethically on a budget, such as buying *either* local *or* organic, growing their own food, purchasing smaller quantities, and shopping at stores that carried alternatives to certified products such as anti-biotic-free meat. We return to these tactics below, but the point to note here is that interviewees with higher incomes appeared most able to obtain ethical foods, describing less tension between their values and their wallets.

Class and income are also connected to community of residence. As noted above, retailers that sell ethical products are typically located in more affluent neighbourhoods. Such is the case in Toronto, where prosperous North Riverdale offers many ethical food choices (especially compared to less affluent South Parkdale), and residents understood their neighbourhood foodscape as directly supporting ethical eating (Johnston, Rodney, and Szabo 2012). Tatjana Radanovic stated, "The whole area of Riverdale is a very good community for farmers' markets, for example. There are enough people with money to buy these things." In contrast, South Parkdale residents had difficulty in accessing appropriate products. Tandy Price, for example, was interested in sustainable fisheries products but couldn't find them locally, except in an "outrageously expensive" health food store. She also noted the cost of taking transit to acquire ethical products: "That's five dollars added on to the price of a piece of salmon."

Like North Riverdale participants, those from Prince Edward County spoke about how effortlessly they acquired ethical foodstuffs. According to Karine Clements, living in the County made it very easy to eat locally. She grew her own food and bought from local organic farmers and vendors, accessing an "amazing" variety. Such ready availability enabled her family's commitment to ethical purchasing and consumption, as did the possession of a garden – something common in rural places such as the County, where many residents have access to arable land. It is worth noting that Prince Edward County and Kingston had higher median incomes than the other sites but had the two lowest costs of living in the study.

Eating habits are also shaped by the food cultures of particular places. If people in a certain environment normally engage in ethical eating, others may feel pressured to follow suit (see Johnston, Rodney, and Szabo 2012). On the other hand, if a person's friends, neighbours, family, and peers are only weakly engaged with ethical eating, and it is not prominent in the local food culture and retail scene, he or she may be less likely to participate in it. For instance, when North Riverdale interviewees were asked to describe a typical eater there, many depicted an idealized, health-conscious, ethical consumer who favoured organic foods. Further, people of varying income levels mentioned feeling a social expectation to live up to this ideal (perhaps by choosing organic raisins for their children's school snacks rather than processed, packaged foods). In the less wealthy and more multicultural neighbourhood of South Parkdale, the dominant version of ethical eating was not strongly established, and participants of all incomes commented on its *lack*. In fact, some seemed only minimally familiar with it.

ENGAGING WITH ETHICAL EATING

Many of the low-income, racialized, and rural families in our sample were weakly or moderately engaged with the dominant ethical eating repertoire (they bought less organic food or knew less about the "buy local" philosophy). For example, of the four racialized immigrant families, three had low engagement and one had moderate engagement. When asked about ethical influences on their eating patterns, they often found the question obscure and confusing – even though they sometimes went on to talk about eating local and "natural" food. Though they may have enacted ethical concerns, their immediate food cultures did not resonate with the ethical eating repertoire.

However, these families cannot be termed "unethical" eaters. Many devoted significant attention to moral dilemmas related to food. Many selected certain aspects of the ethical eating repertoire, adapting them to suit their needs. Others referred to cultural repertoires that fell outside the dominant one. Some of these participants engaged in the same practices as the ideal-typical ethical eater but for different reasons. Sometimes people subscribed to alternative ethical eating repertoires, with different underlying moral frameworks. We observed three patterns among the less involved participants: creative adaptation, alternative moral frameworks, and local loyalties.

Creative Adaptation

Interviewees who employed creative adaptation reconfigured the dominant ethical eating discourse to fit their material circumstances. They were familiar with key tenets of the discourse but had limited access to ethical foods because of their low income. Some focused less on what they bought and cited waste reduction and recycling as evidence of their ethical standing. For example, Taylor Ronald (fifty-five, white, working poor/impoverished), a single mother, stated that she cared about "ethical things" but just couldn't afford to buy organic or fair-trade items. She ate organic food if it was available from her local food bank, or if it was on sale for a very low price. Unable to fully participate in ethical eating through shopping, she and her daughter, Tisha (eighteen), focused on conscientious disposal of food packaging and producing little waste. Tisha took care to recycle, and Taylor mentioned using a Brita filter instead of water bottles and milk bags instead of jugs. She also reduced waste by buying from the bulk food store. She and Tisha saw their minimal consumption – due to low income – as a way to enact care and concern for the environment. These are explicitly ethical food practices, though far less costly than eating organic or adhering to the hundred-mile diet.

Tammy Raikatuji (forty-seven, Japanese Canadian, lower middle class), whose income had been reduced by divorce, also creatively adapted the ethical eating repertoire. She emphasized "not being wasteful" and was deeply concerned about needlessly discarding food. She went to great lengths to use ingredients that were about to expire, which produced some interesting meals, such as a supper of "leftover Kraft Dinner stir-fry with rapini and chili sauce." She could not afford organic meat or dairy products, but she valued sustainability "on a day-to-day living kind of basis." To be clear, participants such as Tammy were highly invested in the dominant mode of ethical consumption and simply found ways to maximize engagement on their limited incomes.

Alternative Moral Frameworks

Some participants employed *alternative* cultural repertoires to engage with moral concerns about eating. Unlike creative adaptation, this strategy was not grounded in the dominant ethical eating repertoire, invoking other frameworks instead.

Alternative approaches, usually connected to ethnicity, were most evident among religious vegetarians. The two Tibetan Canadian families in our sample invoked cultural and religious discourses when describing their moral concerns about eating animals. Although many Euro-Canadians also mentioned restricting meat consumption, most referred to health benefits, environmental impact, or the mistreatment of animals. In contrast, the Tibetan Canadians spoke in terms of culture, religion, and a fundamental relationship to living beings. For instance, Tara Pasang (forty-five, Tibetan Canadian, working class), the mother of three boys, wanted to diminish her meat consumption because "when you grow older, you start thinking more about a religious point of view." Her family was not fully vegetarian, but she followed the Tibetan Buddhist practice of not eating small animals such as shrimp or more than one type of meat per meal. As she put it, "We consider [it] as a sin ... because [it means] eating so many lives at one time." For her fifteen-year-old son, Tenzing, being vegetarian also employed a religious, ethno-cultural repertoire. When asked why he had once tried to be a vegetarian, he said, "I'm Tibetan and we are supposed to; you're not really supposed to eat animals."

In a few cases, participants linked their food practices with moral-ethical issues of poverty and food scarcity in their neighbourhood. Interestingly, only those who had low incomes or had used food banks made this connection. For example, Tanya Pearce (forty-nine, Dutch Canadian, lower middle class), a low-income single mother, patronized a local cafe because it hired at-risk youth and taught them "some life skills, employability skills." This stance was explicitly ethical. In South Parkdale, Trina Parker (fifty-eight, white, working poor/impoverished) spoke about the benefits of the free meals offered by neighbourhood social organizations, "because there's a lot of people that need them." Some lower-income and racialized participants also cooked or shopped for elderly neighbours who needed help – again, plainly ethical concerns. Trina, who received income assistance and struggled to make ends meet herself, had invited "two elderly men who live alone" to share Christmas dinner at her home, "because they have no family." Similarly, Tara Pasang did weekly grocery shopping for some elderly acquaintances. When asked whether ethical issues influenced their eating practices, neither she nor Trina cited their assistance to neighbourhood seniors. Yet the food needs of community members were obviously an ethical concern, and helping seniors enabled them to constitute themselves as moral, caring people. Perhaps the dominant ethical eating repertoire, with its rather limited scope, enjoys such hegemony that other practices are not perceived as ethical – if it's not about local and organic, it doesn't really count.

Local Loyalties

As mentioned above, the dominant discourse asserts that buying local benefits the environment because the food travels shorter distances, reducing greenhouse gases and fuel consumption. Another less common theme is that it supports local farmers and the local economy. This idea was prevalent in interviews with Torontonians, which is not surprising since dominant discourses typically originate in the urban areas that are hubs of media and information dissemination.

Participants from Kingston and Prince Edward County were less engaged with the dominant environmentally focused understanding of eating locally and did not see local eating as primarily a way to improve sustainability. They did connect it with the rural economy, but not in the *abstract,* as was the case in Toronto. Being rural or semi-rural residents themselves, many people in Prince Edward County and Kingston purchased food from family members, neighbours, or friends who were farmers or producers. In addition, buying local was often their most convenient way to shop, and those who lived near the food producers (such as farms that operated roadside stands) talked about the importance of supporting and building relationships with them, who were often their literal or metaphorical neighbours. For these interviewees, buying local was more linked with tradition, mutual support, and even survival than with satisfying an abstract environmental principle. We do not claim that their approach was not ethical, simply that it was not based in the dominant repertoire. Rural and semi-rural participants associated ethical eating with rural dimensions of morality or taking care of the people in their community (Lamont 2000). We describe this as an ethos of "local loyalties," which is socially motivated to support food producers who are often personally known to consumers. The ethos is not entirely separate from the dominant repertoire, but its emphasis on supporting community members differs distinctly from the dominant repertoire's focus on environmental issues.

Trust and localized nationalism were important aspects of the local loyalties ethos. Rural residents believed that locally grown food was safe, superior, and more trustworthy than food from faraway, unknown places, and they exhibited pride in it. Their personal relationships with producers allowed them to access food at what they felt was an affordable price – in contrast to urban interviewees, who complained about cost – and to ask about how it was grown. For example, Keira Karsten (thirty-two, white, working class) emphasized the importance of knowing where food came from and who had produced it:

> I like knowing food came from Prince Edward County, fresh picked this morning, as opposed to not knowing where it came from at all. The kids can go in and pick special, different things. It's interaction with people and with the actual farmers. The kids get to talk to the farmers, try different things and they're more involved. It's about connection.

Likewise, Kristi Keller (thirty-nine, white, working poor/impoverished) appreciated the fact that she could ask questions of the farmers, such as, "What did you use [to grow this]? What's in your soil?" In both Kingston and Prince Edward County, interviewees talked about trusting foods from local sources because they personally knew the producer. Some also believed that Canadian food production standards were superior to those of other countries. Karla Cleveland (forty-two, white, upper middle class) described her aversion to eating food of unknown origin:

> I try to buy local because I want to support my local economy for one. I think the food is better quality, and I know where it comes from. I might know the farmer whose maple syrup we're eating, or I know that farmer whose strawberries we're eating, so I prefer to eat that way if I can than to buy something made in Chile. I probably wouldn't even bother buying it, 'cause it's just from too far away and I have no idea where it's been. And that doesn't feel good.

Here we see that, for people in rural Ontario, "eating local" was often synonymous with consuming food produced by a trusted community member. Such food was seen as superior and less risky than long-distance alternatives, and eating local reflected community pride connected to the rural landscape. Though ethical in nature, it was not motivated primarily by an intellectual impetus to protect the environment.

CONCLUSION

If we accept that shopping and eating to "make a difference" represent a significant way of addressing social and environmental problems, determining how people engage with it is a worthwhile exercise. We found that social position and geographic location affected the ability to take part in the ideas and practices of ethical eating. People from varied class positions, racial-ethnic backgrounds, and urban and rural locations understood ethical eating differently.

For example, economic and cultural capital was strongly connected to the dominant ethical eating repertoire, as socio-economic privilege facilitated access to it (Adams and Raisborough 2010). However, privilege neither guaranteed nor was necessary for strong engagement: some middle-class families (many with high incomes) were weakly engaged, whereas some low-income families had a strong connection.

For some participants, ethical eating differed from the simplistic, market-driven definition that equates "ethics" with access to certain products – a stance that posits low-income eaters as ethically disengaged. Less privileged groups employed creative adaptation and alternative repertoires to consume ethically. Our research thus adds empirical weight to Guthman's (2003, 2008) refutation of the notion that lower-class and racialized people do not connect with moral issues surrounding eating. This point is important, given the history of imputing moral deficiencies to marginalized groups (Schwartz 2000) and the tendency to straightforwardly link ethical consumption with upper-class practices.

Although people can select or reject any element of the ethical eating repertoire, engagement is affected by cultural and economic resources that are inequitably distributed. Ultimately, the repertoire is part of a set of food-related movements and discourses that establish or bolster social hierarchies among people, based on notions of morality (Biltekoff 2013).

3

cosmopolitan eating

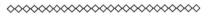

The Vernon Family

THE VERNONS ARE a white, upper-middle-class family of four who live in British Columbia. Their northeast Vancouver neighbourhood is a mix of residences and businesses, as well as income levels. Nearby Commercial Drive, a street lined with multi-ethnic businesses, is a retail centre. Belva (fifty) is originally from New Zealand but has lived in Canada for several decades. She works as a dietitian, which influences the high level of food awareness in her family. Her husband, Brent (fifty-three), is an architect; their annual income exceeds $140,000. Their two sons, Boyd (sixteen) and Blake (fourteen), are in high school. Despite their busy professional lives, the parents make time to prepare home-cooked meals. Food is important to the Vernons, who pride themselves on cosmopolitan eating. Belva handles most of the daily food provisioning, including grocery shopping and meal preparation, but Brent

· · · · · · · · · · · · · · · ·

This chapter was co-authored with Sarah Cappeliez.

regularly bakes bread for the family. He uses a brick oven that he built in the yard, modelled on ones he saw in Greece.

The Vernons are comfortable with cosmopolitan food culture and with European food cultures in particular. Throughout their interviews, they casually referred to cultural eating habits, mentioning that Spanish lunches are longer than North American ones, that Italian children learn to eat vegetables by using olive oil and coarse salt as a dipping sauce (a preparation they themselves used for a dinner party they held), and that Spanish olive oils taste peppery compared to the smoother Italian versions.

The Vernons use their knowledge to distinguish between types of cuisines or food qualities. They love all kinds of restaurants. A favourite French restaurant is described not just as French, but as Alsatian. Another restaurant offers "distinctly flavoured chutneys" and is not "quintessential Indian," but rather fusion in style – a comment recognizing the differences between "authentic" foods and hybrid cuisines. For Belva and Brent, it is extremely important that their sons learn to love cosmopolitan eating. Fourteen-year-old Blake, however, is somewhat uncertain about exotic or unfamiliar restaurants and is hesitant about foods that he does not recognize.

Belva, who is confident in cooking all kinds of cuisines, has taken "serious amateur" courses at an international culinary school in Vancouver and pores over her "vast library" of food magazines and books. Brent also emphasizes the importance of books that help him understand foods and cuisines. He displayed a photograph that he took, in which his favourite French cheeses were artfully arranged beside an encyclopedia entry on cheese. As his photo indicates, he derives pleasure from learning about the foods he enjoys. On the whole, the Vernons present themselves as food connoisseurs, with considerable expertise regarding the markers of authenticity.

··· *The Parker Family*

THE PARKERS ARE a white, working poor/impoverished family of two who live in a densely populated area full of high-rises, in South Parkdale. Tegan Parker (thirteen) lives with her grandmother Trina (fifty-eight) in a one-bedroom government-subsidized apartment. Income constraints shape their engagement with cosmopolitan eating. Trina is unemployed, and they live on an annual income of less than $10,000. She and Tegan have experienced a number of difficulties. In particular, Tegan has bounced between several homes and schools, and thus life concerns loom larger for her than food issues. In spite of struggles with food insecurity, the Parkers are interested in and involved with cosmopolitan eating, in part because of their multicultural surroundings and community experiences that have exposed them to various cuisines.

Trina thoroughly enjoys different kinds of "ethnic" foods as well as learning about them through people in her social network.* *Ackee,* a Caribbean specialty, is her favourite breakfast food. She says, "The one food I don't prefer the most is the basic North American food." She associates North American eating with a "meat and potatoes" style. Unfortunately, low income affects her capacity to purchase cosmopolitan foods, such as ackee and curried goat, because of their prohibitive prices.

For Trina, openness to cosmopolitan foods is intimately tied to community connections. In a previous job, she worked with a diverse immigrant clientele, which exposed her to differing eating habits and shaped her own practices: "I learned a lot through that [job], about different types of foods." Trina's cosmopolitan interests extend to cultural practices and worldviews more broadly. She finds cultural differences "just so fascinating," saying, "It's something worth knowing if you can know a little bit about them all." She also notes the xenophobia and racism that many immigrants face; after she spent time with Muslim friends and adopted their cultural habit of eating with the hands, her boyfriend berated her, calling the habit "piggish." Trina herself, in fact, expresses concern about food safety and hygiene in relation to some ethnic food stores or restaurants, which had sometimes influenced her receptivity to tasting food offered to her by immigrant clients.

Nonetheless, Trina is just as enthusiastic about the injera bread made by an Ethiopian friend as about the wonton soup served at a local bar. She did not discuss whether these foods were made authentically or represented the "best" versions. She enjoys cosmopolitan foods but doesn't seek out food experiences in a systematic way. In short, the Parkers engage in a pragmatic cosmopolitan eating that is facilitated by their multicultural neighbourhood and feasible on a low income.

. . . .

* We apply "ethnic" to foods that come from ethno-cultural traditions outside the Anglo-European mainstream. We recognize the problematic Eurocentricity of this term at the outset.

· · · *The Weaver Family*

NICOLA WEAVER (THIRTY-THREE), a white single mother, lives with her five children in rural Kings County, Nova Scotia. A full-time student at a community college, she makes $16,000 a year. Her eldest daughter, Naeve (fifteen), is home schooled. The Weavers have more limited access to cosmopolitan foods and restaurants than families who live in urban areas. Naeve mentions two "culture restaurants" in their town, which tend to offer "Canadian" versions of Chinese and Mexican dishes. Nonetheless, she recognizes and has tasted some items from other ethnic cuisines, such as butter chicken, and sushi from the local grocery store. Global culture has reached their rural town, and the Weavers are interested in moving beyond the familiar. However, when they have a chance to try more "exotic," unusual, or unfamiliar foods, their general tendency is to hesitate.

For the Weavers, there are more barriers than enablers to experiencing and enjoying cosmopolitan foods and restaurants. Dishes that look "too spicy," such as roti and Indian thali, are not appealing to Nicola, and she is unsure about trying something that she does not recognize: "I don't like eating things when I don't know what it is." For both Nicola and Naeve, eating with one's hands at an Ethiopian restaurant or reaching into several dishes at an Indian restaurant are obstacles. At the same time, ethnic dishes or spaces that recall familiar foods and surroundings are more appealing. For example, injera bread reminds Naeve of a taco, a favourite food among the Weavers, and prompts more enthusiasm than hummus does, which looks like "cat puke" (Naeve) or "unnatural hamburger" (Nicola). Nicola also speaks very positively about a photo of an Ethiopian restaurant, commenting that its decor "looks like home" and that the food looks like something she would try; ultimately, though, she "would be more of a fish and chips girl" when ordering in a restaurant.

Nicola is generally happy with her cooking, although she says she could be more adventurous in incorporating "foreign different spices." She suggests that her tendency to stay with what she knows limits her children's eating experiences and exposure to different tastes. Stir-fries and tacos are staples in the Weaver household, and the family sometimes goes out for donairs or pizza. Such familiar versions of ethnic dishes are viewed as more palatable than foods such as sushi, with nori seaweed that Nicola likens to plastic.

The Weavers display some knowledge of ethnic cuisines – Nicola knows that roti is spicy and that Ethiopian food would be eaten with the hands.

However, her familiarity is limited and not as specific as that of the Vernons or Parkers. For example, in mentioning the chef who prepares sushi at the local supermarket, Naeve describes him as either "Chinese" or "Japanese"; his exact ethnicity is irrelevant, because she believes "he knows more of what he's doing than any of us." Issues of authenticity are absent from her discussion of ethnic foods.

The Weavers, and Naeve especially, show some openness to cosmopolitan eating. Naeve would like to try Indian and Japanese cuisines, and talks about making Japanese food to impress guests, referring to it as to "her taste." Finally, Nicola mentions with pride that Naeve is very good at using chopsticks, which Naeve confirms. The Weavers are thus open to integrating some different foods into their culinary repertoire, as long as they remain within the realm of the somewhat familiar.

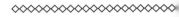

THE THREE FAMILIES presented above hint at what we mean by "cosmopolitan." Cosmopolitanism is generally understood as a disposition and an aptitude to embrace cultural differences. It is most often attributed to classes that have the necessary resources to travel and to take a leisurely interest in the cultures of others (Binnie et al. 2006). It is strongly associated with the mobile and worldly upper classes, yet as Lamont and Aksartova (2002) show, there is reason to believe that other socio-economic and cultural groups engage with it, albeit differently. Cosmopolitan culture is now integral to the daily experiences of people who live in large cities (Devadason 2010). One need not travel extensively to encounter elements of distant cultures, as global culture has infiltrated everyday life. At the same time, differing classes and social groups still express and experience cosmopolitanism in various ways: some people travel the world, sampling diverse cuisines in high-end restaurants, whereas others are exposed to ethnic fare through supermarket sushi and low-priced falafel.

In this chapter, we argue for moving away from a dichotomous characterization that juxtaposes cosmopolitan and non-cosmopolitan. Instead, we suggest that cosmopolitanism itself can be productively understood as a kind of cultural repertoire (Swidler 1986, 2001). Despite the permeability and movement of cultures, it nonetheless operates as a taste hierarchy like other cultural taste hierarchies (Bourdieu 1984).

THEORETICAL FRAMING

Food is an ideal vehicle for studying the lived experience of cosmopolitanism because it stands at the crossroads of daily sustenance and cultural identity. Just as everyday national identity can be expressed through food, everyday cosmopolitanism can be exhibited via the choices that involve culinary conversations across boundaries of nation and ethnicity (Johnston, Baumann, and Cairns 2009). Ordinary people use various types of cosmopolitanism to bridge differences between themselves and others (Lamont and Aksartova 2002; Duruz 2005).

We define cosmopolitan eating as connoting a heightened interest in engaging with varied cuisines outside the Canadian mainstream, with its historic focus on Anglo-Canadian "white bread" and "meat and potatoes" dishes. Cosmopolitan eating involves a multiplicity of practices (such as preparing Indian food at home or shopping at an Asian supermarket) and a range of knowledge (such as recognizing the differences between French cheeses).

Cosmopolitanism, then, is not an orientation that one either possesses or lacks. As a kind of cultural repertoire, it can be creatively employed in daily interactions. Cosmopolitan ideas and experiences are cultural tools, widely sought out, discovered, and referenced through routine food practices. Though not inevitable or universally available, they are employed diversely across classes and rural and urban food environments.

Taste preferences are connected to class divisions, traditionally through "high-brow" foods for elites and "low-brow" foods for the masses (Bourdieu 1984). In contemporary times, this is complicated by omnivorous patterns – consuming widely across high-brow and low-brow genres (Peterson and Kern 1996; Bellavance, Valex, and Ratté 2004; Ollivier 2008). The omnivore now enjoys premier cultural status, having displaced the high-brow snob, who focused solely on elevated culture (such as the opera). In food terms, this means that high-status eaters may possess detailed knowledge of classical French cooking but will also know where to find the most authentic taco stand or an exciting Japanese noodle bar. Omnivorousness and cosmopolitanism are not identical, but they do overlap. To put it simply, omnivorousness entails consumption in differing social status levels, whereas cosmopolitanism focuses on a variety of ethnic cultures, within national boundaries and beyond.

Through choosing authentic exotic foods, eaters may attain status and distinction while simultaneously avoiding the appearance of snobbery (Johnston and Baumann 2010). Authenticity is a notoriously thorny concept, but it commonly involves foods that connect to a certain geographic location, historical production practice (preferably non-industrialized, hands-on, and artisanal), and consumption by a certain ethno-cultural group. Exoticism grants high status to foods that are rare, difficult to obtain, and produced through unique methods (such as small-batch heritage cheeses made by a remote hill people who keep a rare breed of goats). In contrast, inauthentic, unexotic foods that are mass-produced, mundane, and unconnected to a specific place (such as breadsticks at a chain Italian restaurant) are disdained in high-status omnivorous culture. In this chapter, we show how certain cosmopolitan eating practices are overlaid with gourmet culture's privileging of exoticism and authenticity, and similarly function as status markers.

In displacing the high-brow snob, omnivorous elites emphasize their willingness to explore and be open to a variety of cultural products (Peterson and Kern 1996; Ollivier 2008). Such openness can serve as a kind of cultural capital that legitimizes elite taste hierarchies (Ollivier 2008). Cosmopolitan tendencies can reflect a sincere interest in experiencing different cultures, but they can also reinforce and naturalize power hierarchies. Cosmopolitan openness is not politically neutral. Constructing and fetishizing the exotic Other has long been a means of reinforcing the dominance of the mainstream (Said 1978). As bell hooks (1992, 21) remarked, the search for the exotic Other can become "spice, seasoning that can liven up the dull dish that is mainstream White culture." Some people may suggest that their openness to diverse cuisines demonstrates their broadmindedness and lack of racism. Yet consuming the exotic Other through food can itself be a form of "culinary colonialism" (Heldke 2003, xv), even as "a willingness to eat the food of Others seems to indicate at least a growing democracy of the palate" (Narayan 1997, 180).

PARTICIPANTS, PLACES, AND APPROACH TO ANALYSIS

This chapter deals with participants who lived in five sites: three were urban (Vancouver, North Riverdale, and South Parkdale), and two were rural (District of Kent and Kings County). The urban sites showcase a wide array of diverse restaurants, food shops, and culinary ingredients, offering cuisines from around the world. For example, South Parkdale is exceptionally multicultural, serving dishes from Jamaica, Tibet, China, Vietnam, and many other countries. Kings County and the District of Kent display significantly less diversity, but awareness of global cuisines is present in varying degrees. Global commodity chains bring foods from around the world to North American supermarkets. To create a homogeneous sample through which to explore the cosmopolitan eating practices of the culturally dominant group, we included only participants with Euro-Canadian backgrounds.

We examined the interview data to determine how diverse foods, cuisines, and dishes figured in the daily lives of participants, and found that distinctions occurred within and across urban and rural areas. These differences entailed the way in which participants became familiar with varied cuisines, the deliberateness of their cosmopolitanism, their interest in authenticity, and their perceptions of ethnocultural Others (how they spoke about "foreign" people, immigrants, and their food cultures). We identified three modes within the larger cosmopolitan repertoire: connoisseur, pragmatic, and tentative.

CONNOISSEUR COSMOPOLITANISM: KNOWLEDGE AND AUTHENTICITY

Connoisseur cosmopolitanism focused on possessing and showcasing specialized knowledge about international foods and practices. Interviewees prioritized the pleasure of learning about cuisines from around the world and placed a high value on novel food experiences, which they actively sought out and sometimes saw as setting them apart from others.

The connoisseur mode has much in common with Bourdieu's (1984) idea of an upper-middle-class "aesthetic disposition," which implies distance from necessity, with aesthetic appreciation and discovery as sources of pleasure. For example, Nina Wilkinson (forty-seven, white, upper middle class) explained why she sought out new kinds of ethnic food: "There's so many different foods out there, why get bored with the old same stuff?" When asked if she would try eating Indian food with her fingers, she focused on pleasure and novelty: "I'd be game for trying it out. Just something fun, right? I haven't done that. I haven't eaten Indian food with my fingers, but I'd be game!" Nina's son, Nils (sixteen), had also learned to take pleasure in unexplored cuisines and cultures. When shown a picture of Korean food, he explained why he would try it: "I don't really know what it is, but I like most foods in general, and I don't know, Koreans seem pretty wise; I think they'd make good food." In stating why he enjoyed sushi, he revealed an aesthetic disposition regarding food: "It was kind of good 'cause it wasn't just eating ... It was kind of stimulating to the mind too."

Significantly, the connoisseur mode was most frequently articulated by the upper-middle-class families. Their access to this mode appeared to generate a high comfort level with many ethnic cuisines – any and all cuisines were potential targets for learning and exploration. This tendency was evident in two upper-middle-class rural families – the Fitzgeralds and the Woods – suggesting that residence in a cosmopolitan city is not a prerequisite for engagement in the connoisseur mode. As Blanche Fitzgerald (forty-six, white, upper middle class) of the District of Kent put it, "I'm not intimidated by any kind of cooking pretty much." Her husband, Burt, who grew up in a Vancouver suburb, added, "We tend to be fairly adventurous and confident in the kitchen ... My mom was pretty adventurous, and we've sort of carried that on [with our son]. We're pretty adventurous in what we try and our interests."

Living in Kings County, the Wood family (introduced in Chapter 1) was also engaged with the connoisseur approach. Nigel Wood (forty-five, white, upper middle class) stated, "We eat anything." He was proud of his daughters' culinary open-mindedness: "We were eating barbequed chicken feet at the dim sum restaurant, and there's no squeamishness. My younger daughter was probably the only kid in the history of [her] school to bring oxtails and sauerkraut in her lunch." All the Woods spoke positively about their weekly "international nights," when they ate dishes from different ethnicities, including homemade haggis. Before moving to rural Nova Scotia, the Woods lived in urban Ontario, which may be where they adopted the connoisseur approach.

Although connoisseurship involves knowledge about diverse global cuisines, European cuisines and knowledge of them were accorded the most authority. Other studies have found that gourmet food culture frequently legitimates weakly exotic foods, positioning them as more desirable than foods that are extremely distant geographically or culturally (Heldke 2003; Johnston and Baumann 2010). Recall that Brent Vernon photographed French cheeses beside an open reference book and dwelled at length on the enjoyment of learning about food.

As an aside, the fact that gender plays an interesting role in the connoisseur mode is already hinted at here. Although most of our adult interviewees were female, men were rather over-represented in the connoisseur repertoire. Burt Fitzgerald and Nigel Wood are two such examples, as is Brent Vernon, who spoke at length about cheese and baking bread in his wood-fuelled oven. Also, Brandon Vessey mentioned taking cooking classes, and Trent Payne prided himself on his exhaustive knowledge of authentic ethnic cuisines. Seven of the eleven men discussed in this chapter engaged in the connoisseur approach, and all seven were upper middle class. Their willingness to highlight their adventurousness, in a cultural climate where men are expected to be "meat-and-potatoes guys" (Sobal 2005), suggests that their masculinity was already assured in other ways related to class (Connell and Messerschmidt 2005), as discussed in Chapter 1. In other words, as upper-middle-class men, they could afford to enact different (or non-dominant) versions of masculinity by displaying an interest in exotic cooking.

Another common connoisseur theme was seeking knowledge from expert sources such as gourmet magazines, cookbooks, websites, and cooking schools. For instance, Trish Rendell (forty-three, white, upper middle class) enrolled in a traditional French cooking class to improve her knowledge and ability to recognize foods in restaurants: "What I wanted was to be able – when I go to a restaurant or somewhere and I taste something and I have no clue how it was made to taste the way that it did, how do they do it?" As mentioned above, Brandon Vessey (fifty-nine, white, upper middle class) took cooking classes "because I wanted to learn how to do French cooking." He took French-language classes simultaneously to enhance the depth of his learning.

Just as familiarity with the connoisseur mode afforded a certain confidence in cosmopolitan eating, the lack of familiarity (such as gaps in knowledge about European food culture) made some individuals feel self-conscious and uncomfortable. This discomfort can be associated with low economic capital (and thus the inability to afford fine dining or cooking classes), but in our sample it was also related to the lack of cultural capital, perhaps linked to living in a somewhat remote rural area. For example, Blanche Fitzgerald (forty-six, white, upper middle class) of the District of Kent connected her discomfort with lack of knowledge: "I have been uncomfortable, once or twice, in expensive restaurants. Because I'm not really a connoisseur of wine and I'm not really sure – and the etiquette, I feel that I should know the etiquette and I don't."

Another key connoisseur trait was an interest in the cuisine of exotic Others, especially foods that were seen as authentic, which usually meant being prepared and enjoyed by people of that ethno-cultural group. The words "interesting" and "fascinating" were commonly used here. The appreciation of authenticity distinguished between versions of the same dish and rejected "inauthentic" mass-produced items that were consumed with minimal thought and knowledge. Finding the "best," "truest," and most legitimate version of a food – a tortilla, roti, or *churrasco* chicken – was an important goal. Trent and Tina Payne (fifty-three and fifty-one, white, upper middle class) demonstrated their ability to recognize authentic versions of ethnic food in discussing a roti shop that Trent dubbed "the best." Tina continued, "It's Guyanese roti, so, different than some of the Caribbean rotis. We've got friends who swear by other roti shops. We're, like, 'No, no, no!'" Nigel and Nanette Wood (forty-five and forty-three, white, upper middle class) described a "horrible" Indian restaurant where everything was microwaved, including the naan bread, which is traditionally prepared in a wood-fired oven: "We asked for fresh naan bread, and it took twenty minutes, and it was microwaved!" In cataloguing the shortcomings of this restaurant, the Woods simultaneously established their own knowledge of authenticity.

In connoisseur cosmopolitanism, consumption ranges broadly across ethnic cuisines but is also highly selective. Commonplace items are less valued than unusual, exotic fare. For example, Nigel Wood noted that "raw fish" and sashimi were preferable to a mundane California roll. He said of butter chicken, "I'd eat that. It's not what I usually order at Indian restaurants, because I'll go for something more exotic."

The emphasis is on finding foods from specific places (Guyanese roti surpasses generic Caribbean roti), and connoisseurs value travelling to various parts of their neighbourhood, city, or even around the world to acquire superior – more authentic and exotic – items. For example, Therese Parsons (forty-five, white, upper middle class) framed her choice to patronize a Latin American shop that sells "real-deal" tortillas as "an example of how I don't just go to the one grocery store. I will look for places even if it's out of my way." Upper-middle-class families in both rural and urban settings linked extensive knowledge about ethnic foods with travelling and/or living abroad. For example, Burt Fitzgerald (forty-three, white, upper middle class) associated his knowledge of Indian foods with his travels in India.

For connoisseur cosmopolitans, knowledge of different ethnic cuisines constitutes the discerning consumer. Knowledge of European canons, of exotic foods, and of authenticity grants distinction in this complex culinary hierarchy. Seeing food as the object of inquiry and the search for authenticity and exoticism as pleasurable conveys an elite distance from necessity (Bourdieu 1984).

PRAGMATIC COSMOPOLITANISM: EXPOSURE THROUGH EXPERIENCE

The pragmatic mode of cosmopolitanism centres on real-world connections with a food culture and its people. This mode is inspired by practical, day-to-day experiences, such as working or living with someone of a different ethno-cultural background – a kind of ethnographic experience. The pragmatic mode was particularly prominent among urban residents and was expressed by interviewees with varying degrees of economic and cultural capital. Pragmatic cosmopolitanism may involve acquiring knowledge about a new food or cuisine, but this is not its motivating rationale. Instead, the mode develops more organically, and unintentionally, prompted by encounters with diverse people and food cultures through everyday life. Displays of this mode establish the individual as a casual, urbane sophisticate rather than an elite world traveller.

Trina Parker's orientation to global foods vividly demonstrates the pragmatic mode, and her story shows that it is not contingent on elite practices. Trina enjoyed living in a diverse multicultural neighbourhood. She spoke eagerly about dishes that spanned several types of cuisines, showing her preference for a non-meat-and-potatoes diet. Her openness to different ways of eating was accompanied by a desire to better understand immigrant worldviews and experiences. Trina exemplifies pragmatic engagement with eating practices and foods that are distant from her own culture, at the same time showing that this mode need not be accompanied by connoisseur elements. Her approach relies more on enthusiasm and openness than on the esoteric knowledge and cultural specificity of the connoisseur mode. For example, she referred to hot Japanese "green paste," forgetting the name wasabi, and she described the spices in a roti generically as "Indian spice," rather than listing them meticulously.

It is important to note that people can display elements of both the connoisseur and pragmatic modes. Although access to cultural repertoires is structured by privilege, these various modes are employed with agency and creativity, in keeping with the idea of cosmopolitanism as a kind of cultural or culinary repertoire. The ethnographic experience is key to the pragmatic mode. For example, Nigel Wood demonstrated many connoisseur tendencies, but he also placed a priority on food *experiences*. He described unintentionally eating horse meat while travelling in Italy as a "fun" experience. Bronwyn Vale (forty-one, white, lower middle class) dreamed of travelling through Mexico to "write the recipes, and their histories and their cultural references and all of that." Although she was interested in food knowledge and recipes, she seemed most passionate about experiencing Mexican culture, which she perceived as exciting and different from her own. In this way, knowledge about foods and cuisines can be acquired through first-hand encounters, rather than from reference books or cooking classes. Here Bronwyn's interest in cosmopolitan consumption speaks more to a desire for novel cross-cultural experiences than to a wish to acquire an encyclopedic knowledge of food.

Pragmatic practices may entail travel experiences but can also be based in local, rooted engagement with food. Participants noted that they could use their neighbourhoods as gateways to global food knowledge. In cities such as Toronto and Vancouver, cosmopolitan ingredients, food stores, and restaurants are widely available. Many immigrant communities live and set up businesses in the culturally diverse neighbourhoods that we studied. Thus, pragmatism could emerge from the exploration and enjoyment of what was readily available and proximate, which meant that it was not limited to those with abundant economic or cultural resources. Tandy Price (forty-nine, European and Middle Eastern, lower middle class) repeatedly emphasized the diversity of restaurants and shops in her South Parkdale neighbourhood. Trina Parker (fifty-eight, white, working poor/impoverished) spoke about several restaurants that she frequented (Caribbean, Chinese, Vietnamese), all in her own neighbourhood, and described her community with pride:

> Basically, anything you feel like eating, you can probably find that type of food here. If you want perogies, I'll take you out to [a nearby street] for a perogy dinner. There's Tibetan here, there's an Ethiopian place, there's Chinese, there's Vietnamese, there's Pizza Pizza, there's Caribbean – there's, like, three roti shops. There's a lot. Anything you want, you can probably get.

This kind of multicultural eating is clearly not as evident, or possible, in rural areas that don't experience transnational flows of culture and people to the same degree. For example, in Kings County, Natalia Warshawski (forty-seven, white, lower middle class) noted that the grocery store did not sell sushi. Others in Kings County were frustrated by the unavailability of diverse cuisines and spices. Beryl Fredericks (thirty-eight, white, lower middle class), in the District of Kent, argued that the transnational friendship networks of urban living enabled exposure to diversity: "You might really like Korean food, because you have had it before or you have friends with a variety of ethnic backgrounds and you have eaten at their houses, so you have expanded more of what you like in general. There is more a chance of that happening, I think, in an urban setting." As suggested by Beryl, the main sources of pragmatic knowledge are not textbooks or experts, but colleagues, neighbours, and the community at large. This was exemplified by Trina's description of discovering ethnic cuisines through interactions with multicultural clients and co-workers who brought food to her former workplace. Once introduced to new foods, Trina "gave up a lot of the other stuff" that she disliked. Similarly, Taylor Ronald (fifty-five, white, working poor/impoverished), who had learned about different cuisines through a Vietnamese neighbour and a women's centre, stated, "You sort of develop a palate. You know, some of it is really good."

For pragmatists, openness to foods and cultures was largely due to daily involvement with diverse communities, which obviously hinged on the accessibility of transnational flows of people, capital, and goods. Lacking this, the pragmatic experience could not occur, and indeed, it was much rarer among residents in the District of Kent and Kings County. Our data suggest that pragmatism is a distinct variety of urban cosmopolitanism, one available even to those with limited resources and minimal geographic mobility. Contrary to the notion that cosmopolitanism is exclusively about the display of cultural capital and status, the pragmatic mode demonstrates the capacity of some urban-dwellers to develop multicultural culinary tastes and to have food experiences beyond their culture of origin.

TENTATIVE COSMOPOLITANISM: AMBIVALENCE

Tentative cosmopolitanism was slightly more prominent among economically marginalized and rural participants, though it was also evident in Toronto and Vancouver. When tentative cosmopolitans sorted pictures of foods into categories with which they were comfortable and uncomfortable, they demonstrated less interest in and familiarity with dishes that were relatively common in Toronto and Vancouver (Indian butter chicken, tacos, falafel, roti, sushi). Beryl Fredericks (thirty-eight, white, lower middle class) suggested that this preference for familiar foods was a "rural thing," where people are less exposed to ethnic cuisines: "If you grow up on a farm or in a logging community or something, you are going to eat more food like that ... more meat-and-potatoes." In eating local (see Chapter 2), rural participants necessarily opted for the familiar – food grown by themselves or their neighbours.

Of course, global food and culture do penetrate rural areas to some extent. For example, in Kings County, Nevada Wheeler (fifteen, white, working poor/impoverished) mentioned making sushi in family studies class, though she stated, "I really, really don't like it ... It was pretty gross." Nicola Weaver (thirty-three, white, working poor/impoverished) described an Indian restaurant in her small town but added, "I don't go there ... I've never gone there." When asked why, she replied, "Well, people say it's really spicy." To be clear, our point is not to "objectively" compare the availability of foods of diverse ethnicities in rural areas or to measure the level of familiarity with them. Our interest is to broadly portray the tentative mode of engagement with ethno-cultural cuisines, assuming, of course, that they were less common in rural districts than in the multicultural neighbourhoods of Toronto and Vancouver.

The tentative mode of engagement is characterized chiefly by ambivalence. Overall, it combines appreciation for tastes that are familiar and close to home with hesitancy about new food experiences from other cultures. It is commonly accompanied by the view that food is a practical necessity rather than a pleasure or an adventure, a disposition usually associated with working-class cultures (Bourdieu 1984). Trudy Patterson (sixty, white, working poor/impoverished) exemplified this attitude regarding food, which she saw as performing a function and not warranting extensive attention: "I cook kind of very simply, like, nothing that uses a whole lot of ingredients or a whole lot of spices, or I don't try new recipes. I'm just not into that. Food is just something to me that's kind of necessary to eat; you try to have something tasty, but it's not, like, huge importance in my life." Trudy linked eating with basic nourishment rather than exploration. As she clearly articulated, food was primarily a necessity, and taste took second place.

Nonetheless, in the tentative mode, encounters with diverse cuisines do occur, almost as an unavoidable result of living in a multicultural country – a kind of culinary osmosis rather than conscious exploration. Beryl Fredericks said this explicitly: "Generally, our culture is moving towards a bit more of an integrated diet. As more people get exposed to all the different ethnic flavours, it's just happening without people even realizing it." Despite her largely functional approach to food, Trudy Patterson stated that her eating habits had changed substantially after she moved to Toronto, with exposure to "the choices that are available." Nonetheless, she expressed more hesitancy than enthusiasm for these changes (see Chapter 7 for her case study). She showed little interest in or attention to the details of the new dishes she had added to her repertoire: "I forget what it's called; there's a name for it. Anyway, it's all lentils and it's spiced and it's on a piece of bread or something or a wrap. But I don't eat them that way, but I should eat more stuff like that."

Trudy showed no desire to prove that she could discern authenticity. In the District of Kent, an exchange between Bree Fagan (fifty-six, Swiss Canadian, lower middle class) and her sixteen-year-old daughter Beata had a similar tone. They described a restaurant they had enjoyed but couldn't remember the ethnicity of its cuisine. They thought it might be Indian, Lebanese, Persian, or perhaps Parisian. A willingness to eat a variety of foods need not make them the focus of attention. Indeed, many tentative cosmopolitans desired to be open to diverse cuisines but were not particularly interested in discovering more about them.

The ambivalence of the tentative approach was also expressed in a reluctance to explore ethno-cultural cuisines. Openness was countered by diffidence. For example, Becky Fanning (thirty-nine, white, working class) was both "leery" of sushi and interested in it: "I haven't tried it. It looks really nice. I'm a little bit leery because I've heard it is raw fish, but like I said, I haven't heard of anybody getting sick or dying from it, so I'd try it." Nicola Weaver (thirty-three, white, working poor/impoverished) voiced the most outright suspicion, but even she expressed an ambivalent willingness to expand her cooking repertoire: "I'm happy with my cooking. I guess I could be a little bit more broader. Like, these foreign different spices or different foods or – I would like to be able to do that, but I get my likes and I stick with it." As we note in Chapter 6, experimenting with new tastes carries much higher risk when finances are limited.

Beryl Fredericks expressed similar ambivalence about expanding her culinary repertoire; the idea of cooking ethnic dishes was appealing, but the practicalities, especially her children's preferences, seemed too daunting:

> I don't think I'm a very experimental cook, and I would like to expand into more foods that are ethnic in origin. Like, I'd like to become an amazing Thai cook or something like that. But it's not a priority right now. Unless I think that my kids are going to like it, I'm probably not going to cook it ... I'm a little bit conservative that way.

Beryl stated that she had raised her children in a "fairly basic North American style," recalling that they had once tried Filipino food but "didn't like it all." She believed that "adults are always looking for a new flavour experience," whereas "kids just want something familiar." This is an interesting contrast to the socialization expectations of connoisseurs, who saw a parent's role as training children's taste buds to appreciate new flavours, open to exploring any and all cuisines. Some rural teenagers agreed with Beryl's view: Noni Webster (eighteen, white, lower middle class) believed that Korean food would probably be eaten only by a teen "who was really, like, cultured, you know?"

Some participants suggested that hesitancy could be overcome through personal connections. Responding to a photo of North Indian thali, Nils Wilkinson (sixteen, white, upper middle class) said, "I don't even know what that is. I wouldn't order that. I'd probably eat it if I was at some North Indian dude's house ... I doubt that would ever happen." He also thought an Ethiopian restaurant looked "kind of weird," stating, "I probably wouldn't eat there unless someone took me there." Tanya Pearce (forty-nine, Dutch Canadian, lower middle class) also suggested that she could be persuaded to try diverse cuisines:

> Some of them definitely look "ethnic," and chances are it would be somebody else suggesting "How about we try this," right? ... I don't know if I would do it totally on my own ... obviously for some of those restaurants or cultures, like, the cultures that maybe I haven't had their food before ... But somebody says, "Hey Tanya, this is really great, let's go" and I'd say "Sure, why not?"

Tanya's openness to unfamiliar food depended on being introduced to it through personal contact. In the tentative mode, this may be an important gateway for exposure to cuisines, particularly when low income makes trying new foods (that the children may refuse) quite impractical.

Although a personal connection could potentially bridge the divide between the familiar and the unfamiliar, the tentative mode sometimes extended to suspicion or skepticism, labelling exotic foods in negative terms – as "unappealing," "awful," or "weird," with dubious edibility. Noni Webster (eighteen, white, lower middle class) described herself as a "proud ... picky eater" who didn't like "a lot of seasoning" and felt that Korean food "just looks gross." Shown a picture of butter chicken, she responded, "I love chicken, but that looks like a baby puked on it. It looks terrible. If you scraped off all the gross and just left the flavour, maybe." Nicola Weaver (thirty-three, white, working poor/impoverished) reacted in a similar fashion to a photograph of Chinese food: "I don't think I would even touch that. It's just not my culture, I guess. I like rice but I don't know a lot about Chinese. I mean, I know I go to Chinese restaurants, but if there is something different there, I won't touch it either." Asked how she might react if a friend recommended a Chinese restaurant, she replied, "What would I say? 'Why would you want to go there?'" Similarly, she would not try Korean food, "because I don't know what it is."

This dismissal of ethnic cuisines was not the dominant view among participants, though it did occur in other interviews, principally with people from rural areas and those whose economic and cultural capital was limited. Trudy Patterson (sixty, white, working poor/impoverished) summed up the lack of interest in discovering new foods: "Unknown ingredients, unknown taste. Not appealing to me. Wouldn't eat 'em." Both Bram Fortuyn (fourteen, white, working class) and Toni Roberts (forty-nine, white, working poor/impoverished) responded simply to images of ethnic food: "It looks too foreign." Notably, all the participants quoted above were low income. Their resistance to cosmopolitan eating (a status marker) could also express differing priorities regarding food, particularly concerning provision of nourishment on a budget.

The tentative mode also emphasized the appeal of traditional, or "Canadian," foods, especially those eaten during youth. Although open to new food, participants were strongly drawn to the tastes of home, the familiar. For example, Toni Roberts talked about adding new ethnic foods to her diet but still seemed to identify strongly with those of her youth: "Basically, I would say that my eating habits are definitely from the way I was brought up." Although she suggested that her diet had broadened, she did not explain how multicultural choices fit into her daily consumption.

The appeal of "home" was also apparent in the preference for familiar North American versions of cosmopolitan foods, such as Chinese Canadian buffets and Italian American pastas, which were seen as more trustworthy, familiar, and less risky. Widely available commercial versions of ethnic foods (such as those served at the Olive Garden chain restaurant) were viewed as more palatable than "authentic" dishes. Naish White (sixteen, Acadian Canadian, working class) and his brother Nelson (thirteen) liked the Chinese food in Kings County because it was "more of a mix of Chinese and Canadian cuisine." They were unimpressed by the Chinese food in Toronto and Calgary: "They're real Chinese food, like, if you went in, like, one in Chinatown in Toronto, most of the Chinese people don't speak English there, they're really, real Chinese food, like, the spicy kinds and the salty fish and sushi and stuff."

CONCLUSION

As it unfolds in everyday life, cosmopolitanism is multi-faceted and complex (Lamont and Aksartova 2002). Our study found important differences between urban and rural engagement with cosmopolitanism and discerned three distinct modes: connoisseur, pragmatic, and tentative. Prioritizing knowledge acquisition and authenticity, the connoisseur mode employed cosmopolitan eating as a source of cultural capital. The pragmatic mode relied on connections built through personal experiences and was not exclusively linked to specialized knowledge. The tentative mode encountered global tastes more by accident than design, though low income and/or rural location could render such contact infrequent. Given the strong connection between high social status and the connoisseur mode, the tentative approach was unlikely to accrue much cultural capital. It featured ambivalence regarding unfamiliar tastes and a desire to stay connected with the tastes of home. In urban areas, connoisseur modes were linked to economic capital, but low-income individuals could also engage in the pragmatic mode. Rural participants were less likely to display this mode, given their more limited exposure to diverse people and cuisines.

These distinctions can help scholars better understand how cosmopolitan values may be enacted by differently privileged groups. Although our analysis showed that cosmopolitanism was not limited to elites, the connoisseur mode did imply a taste hierarchy and mapped onto hierarchies associated with gourmet food cultures that value authenticity and exoticism (Johnston and Baumann 2010). Connoisseur cosmopolitans with substantial economic and cultural resources prized an exotic culinary Otherness as intellectually interesting and fun (Heldke 2003). Those with less disposable income and fewer cultural resources could view the foods of the Other more cautiously, even negatively. Familiar dishes were often privileged over unfamiliar ones, in part because there was less financial, cultural, or taste risk involved in consuming them.

4

vegetarian eating

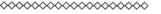

The Pasang Family

THE PASANGS ARE a Tibetan Canadian, low-income, working-class family who live in South Parkdale, which is home to many Tibetan Canadian families, as well as restaurants and stores selling Tibetan food. Tara Pasang (forty-five) and Tseten Pasang (forty-five) immigrated to Canada from India six years ago with their three sons. Tara is a personal support worker, and Tseten is a bookkeeper; their annual income is about $30,000. Their two youngest sons, Tenzing (fifteen) and Thekchen (nine), attend local public schools. Their eldest son, Tsering (twenty), now lives in India, having moved there to join a monastery as a Buddhist monk.

The Pasangs' three-bedroom apartment is in a building that houses many other Tibetan Canadian families. They eat primarily Tibetan and Indian food prepared at home by Tara. She and Tseten make the decisions regarding the purchase and consumption of food, and the family eats most meals at home, except for the occasional visit to a local Tibetan restaurant. Tara's primary

. . . .

This chapter was co-authored with Alexandra Rodney.

concerns are that food be fresh and that her children do not eat too many frozen or prepackaged items, which she considers "junk food." Tenzing sees Tara and Tseten as "typical Asian parents" who decline his involvement in decisions about food, although Tara does try to engage him in the kitchen by assigning small tasks such as chopping vegetables.

Both children, Tenzing and Thekchen, would prefer a wider variety of food, particularly more "Western" foods. Tenzing would also like to have more say in what the family eats. He converted to vegetarianism for a few months, in accordance with his Buddhist faith, but family tensions associated with this move prompted him to revert to meat. As a Tibetan Buddhist, Tenzing says, "You're not really supposed to eat animals." Whereas eldest brother Tsering is a vegetarian, the rest of the family eats meat.

Eating with other Tibetans is important to the Pasangs, who often share food and meals with friends and relatives, many of whom live nearby. Social gatherings tend to centre on meat-based Tibetan dishes, and as Tenzing mentioned, avoiding meat is a particular challenge at such times.

As we saw in Chapter 2, Tara is becoming more interested in religious dictates regarding food and thus seeks to eat less meat: "When you grow older, you start thinking more about a religious point of view." Nonetheless, Tenzing feels that she was unsupportive of his vegetarian aspirations: "I tried to be a vegetarian for, like, two or three months, and it didn't quite work out so well because me and my mom kind of had arguments." In particular, Tara found it difficult to make separate meals for him or meatless meals others would eat. In spite of "feeling guilty as a Buddhist" for eating meat, Tara says, "For dinner, we eat meat most of the time. Chicken or beef. I don't feel like eating something without meat. I feel unsatisfied." She is also concerned about the healthfulness of vegetarianism, fearing that Tenzing will not get enough iron from a meatless diet. Clearly, some teens face challenges within and outside the family when they adopt vegetarianism.

··· The Rendell Family

THE RENDELLS ARE a white, high-income, upper-middle-class family who live in North Riverdale. Trish (forty-three) and Tom (forty-two), who are both high-school teachers, share the cooking duties. Daughters Tai (thirteen) and Tannis (nine) make their own breakfast, lunch, and after-school snacks. Despite the family's income (about $110,000, not too far above the community median), the Rendells shop at discount food stores and make most of their food at home. Eating out is a treat. Trish, who taught high-school nutrition at one point, describes the family's goal as "eating real food," as opposed to packaged foods, and otherwise aiming to eat a balanced diet by following Canada's Food Guide. The family still leaves room for indulgent foods, though, because, as Trish says, "They just taste good!"

Weekday work commitments affect the amount of time that Trish and Tom can devote to evening meals. Their strategy to address this challenge is to spend their Sundays making several meals that will be reheated during the week. Because they enjoy a variety of flavours, they prepare dishes from many ethnic cuisines (such as curries). Tom and Trish contribute equally to advance-meal preparation, although Trish jokes that Tom is a little more absent-minded in regard to cooking: "He doesn't mind if the food is a little burnt." She also notes, "He doesn't read the instructions or food labels."

Despite claiming that she lacks a "flair" for cooking, Trish describes herself as "addicted to shopping for kitchen gadgets on eBay." She collects cook-books and allocates much of her weekend to grocery shopping and preparing weekday dinners for the family. She also received a French cook-ing certificate from a local college. Trish would like to eat "food that is low on the food chain," referring to both plant-based and unprocessed items.

Both Trish and Tom became vegetarians during university, a decision that Trish describes as being sparked by a desire to eat food that was "more inter-esting" than the dishes made by her mother, who "wasn't a good cook." When they realized that the demands of being graduate students had led them to a "Diet Coke and French fry" version of vegetarianism, the Rendells began to eat more meat. Trish still avoids red meat and often chooses vegetarian options.

Their daughter Tai has been a vegetarian for about three years, a decision she made for ethical reasons. She thinks it's not "fair to the animals" to kill them for food. She was inspired to become a vegetarian after her exposure to environmental and ethical teachings at an "eco-camp," and has been en-couraged by a vegetarian family friend who is something of a mentor for her. Tai's conversion to vegetarianism did not cause tension in the family. Trish and Tom respect and accommodate her preference by making either a nightly vegetarian meal for the whole family or a separate one that Trish shares with Tai. The Rendells appear to seamlessly adjust their meal planning and prep-aration to respect the preference of their teenage daughter.

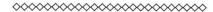

THIS CHAPTER FOCUSES on teen vegetarianism and its impact on family eating habits and emotional dynamics. During their teenage years, many people experiment with vegetarianism in expressing an ethical and/or healthy eating style. In Chapter 1, we examined how vegetables are understood as the cornerstone of healthy eating, not least because they may aid in reducing or maintaining body weight. Engagement with healthy eating varies by gender and age. In Chapter 2, we explored how ethical eating entailed the expression of moral or political values through food choices. Opting not to eat meat may be grounded in ethical beliefs concerning animal rights and the environment.

When teens become vegetarians, what is revealed through their choice and the responses of family members, concerning the intersection of class and gender in family food practices? We analyzed the interview data from all 105 families across Canada, selecting those in which vegetarianism was discussed. We used a broad definition of "vegetarian," including anyone who self-identified as such, regardless of whether they ate fish, dairy, or eggs, since vegetarian diets differ so widely (Barr and Chapman 2002). In total, forty-six participants identified as current or former vegetarians, twenty-two of whom were teenagers.

THEORETICAL FRAMING

Choices about vegetarianism intersect with existing social hierarchies and do not occur in a vacuum. In Western countries, vegetarians tend to be female, upper-middle-class, highly educated, white teenagers or young adults (Perry et al. 2001; Ruby 2012). Reasons for becoming a vegetarian vary but are most commonly related to health, body image, and ethics (Lacobbo and Lacobbo 2006; Fox and Ward 2008; Greene-Finestone et al. 2008). A vegetarian identity is not static – vegetarians can return to meat eating, and meat-eaters can become vegetarians at differing times throughout their lives (Barr and Chapman 2002; Menzies and Sheeshka 2012).

The fact that most who self-identify as vegetarian are female resonates with dominant perceptions that meat is masculine, as seen in Chapter 1 (Sobal 2005). Meat is associated with men's higher status in patriarchal societies, the hunting and killing of animals is traditionally done by men, and meat is thought to signify strength and power over other beings. Consequently, a man's decision to eat meat can be seen as a display of masculinity (Brownlie and Hewer 2007). At the same time, vegetarianism tends to be perceived as healthy eating, which, as discussed in Chapter 1, is understood as a feminine purview (Ruby 2012). Thus, it is not surprising that girls and women are significantly more likely to consider or adopt vegetarianism, whether for health or ethical reasons (ibid.).

Social class also shapes vegetarian eating. Seemingly simple choices – whether to eat a hamburger or a falafel – depend not only on individual preferences but also on the cultural and material resources that constrain or enable dietary choices. As mentioned in Chapters 2 and 3, cultural theorists note that food decisions are affected not simply by individual proclivities, but also by cultural skills, knowledge, and beliefs (Swidler 1986). Perceiving taste as part of collective culture enables us see that vegetarianism may cluster with other classed taste preferences, such as particular modes of cosmopolitan or ethical eating. Those who enjoy greater class privilege may be better positioned to pay considerable attention to food concerns beyond simply meeting their basic needs (Bourdieu 1984; Johnston and Baumann 2010). There is even some indication that upper-middle-class men may establish their masculinity so convincingly through other means that dispensing with meat eating is relatively risk-free for them and is perhaps even an expected part of their healthy or stylish eating (Rimal 2002; Gossard and York 2003).

When teens become vegetarians, a potential for family conflict arises (Lacobbo and Lacobbo 2006). Parents may perceive the change as a rejection of their eating style, and given the emphasis on meat and masculinity, fathers may be particularly antagonistic (Roth 2005; Merriman 2010). Parents can pressure or challenge teens to eat meat and can refuse to accept dietary change. With women taking responsibility for most of a family's foodwork (Beagan et al. 2008), accommodating a vegetarian can add significantly to their labour, as was the case for Tara Pasang. Nonetheless, mothers tend to be more accepting than fathers of teen vegetarianism (Ruby 2012). Not surprisingly, those with greater social support are more likely to maintain vegetarian diets (Barr and Chapman 2002; Cherry 2006).

PARTICIPANTS, PLACES, AND APPROACH TO ANALYSIS

For this chapter, we selected all participants who self-identified as vegetarian. These included twenty-six people who had once been vegetarian (nine of whom were teens) and twenty who were currently vegetarian (thirteen teens). Fourteen of the twenty-two teens were girls and eight were boys; sixteen came from middle-class families, and six were from working-class or impoverished families. (Interestingly, among the adults, all former and current vegetarians were from middle-class families.) Most participants had adopted vegetarianism for ethical motives, though adults were more likely to do so for health reasons.

In our sample, female vegetarian teens outnumbered their male counterparts, as predicted by the literature, but one-third of the group was nonetheless male. This does not necessarily mean that the gendering of vegetarian eating is changing, with more boys adopting it. It is equally possible that the male teens who were willing to talk about food were particularly interested in it – traditionally a feminine domain. They may have been disproportionately likely to be interested in vegetarian eating, for health or ethical reasons. To be clear, though, similar proportions of boys and girls were vegetarian.

To determine how people viewed vegetarian eating, we carefully examined all instances in which they spoke about their own vegetarianism (current or past), or about vegetarianism in the abstract. We paid specific attention to teenagers' experiences with vegetarianism and how these related to parental attitudes and family dynamics.

We categorized all the families in which there was at least one former or current teen vegetarian (sixteen families) as either "supportive" or "resistant." The vast majority (thirteen) were supportive. At the time of the interviews, the teens in ten of the thirteen supportive families had maintained their vegetarianism, and some had done so for several years. The supportive families had a range of income and class levels, but there was a clear link to class. Only three were from lower-class backgrounds; all three were headed by single mothers who were well educated but whose income was low due to divorce or disability (see Chapter 6 for a discussion of class change and food practices).

In the three resistant families, none of the teens maintained their meatless diets for more than a few months. All the resistant families were low income and were either working class or working poor/impoverished. Caution is warranted, however, concerning the class implications here. There were only 3 families out of 105 in which parents actively resisted teen vegetarianism. The data are at best suggestive of class patterns.

VEGETARIANISM AND CULTURAL REPERTOIRES

Our data indicate that parents drew from their own cultural repertoires in accepting or rejecting their teenager's vegetarianism. Some
repertoires made accommodation seem easy or even effortless. For
example, many middle-class parents had extensive cooking skills
and knew where to find and how to prepare "exotic" ingredients (see
Chapter 3) and meat substitutes. Support was also linked to their
broader cultural tool kits – such as information gathering, product
research, and other shopping skills – that could be employed to accommodate teen vegetarianism. Such skills are not exclusive to middle-
class parents, but they are a particular form of cultural capital that
attaches to class.

Some of the more supportive parents had once been vegetarians
themselves and could thus refer to a pre-existing repertoire – the
necessary shopping, cooking, and eating strategies were already in
their tool kits (Swidler 1986), though perhaps a little rusty. These parents talked with relative ease and nonchalance about their child's
adoption of vegetarianism and the resultant need to purchase or prepare different foods. They were also unencumbered by fears about
vegetarianism and health. Ted Rodger (fifty-two, white, upper middle
class), who had a strong belief in the benefits of healthy eating, felt
that making meatless meals for Ty, his sixteen-year-old son, was not
a burden: "His mother had been a vegetarian; I was a vegetarian in
university. So it wasn't really a big shift for us to do that; it was quite
accommodating. And also, we understood how healthy it was, and it
was good for us." In fact, supportive parents (both those who had
been vegetarians and those who had not) saw the omission of meat as
a particularly healthy life choice.

Even parents who had no vegetarian cooking skills summoned
elements from their broader culinary repertoires. Trish Rendell (pro-
filed above) drew from her extensive knowledge of cooking to accommodate both the vegetarians and non-vegetarians in her family. She
talked about making a meal that met everyone's needs:

> If we have something like butter chicken, a common meal on our
> roster, we do a tofu route as well. So the same sauce, but with
> tofu. And for Tai, we get the veggie chicken. It's like a tofu
> chicken but looks like chicken slices. We scoop out the butter

chicken sauce and warm up the veggie chicken slices in that. So Tai can get all the pleasure of the flavour without eating the chicken.

Supportive parents also mobilized information-gathering skills to expand their culinary offerings. Through her work in a health clinic, Nuala Haldane (forty, white, working class) was familiar with using food to promote a healthy lifestyle, and though she had never been a vegetarian, she felt confident in her ability to expand her knowledge via the Internet. Before her fourteen-year-old daughter Nikki became a vegetarian, Nuala depended on her usual meat-based recipes. Afterward, she frequently searched the Internet for recipes and cooking instructions: "I've been going on the Internet, getting recipes off a vegetarian place. They have lots of them on there. The Internet's a great place for recipes. So I've been doing that and trying to cook those recipes for her. I made raisin orange couscous the other day, and I made sesame seed pasta."

Resistant families were generally less familiar with vegetarian repertoires. Because empirically documenting the absence of a repertoire is difficult, we investigated attitudes regarding vegetarian eating in our broader (non-vegetarian) sample that might help explain how and why it was rejected or discredited. Some participants who seemed uninterested in vegetarianism also displayed little interest in food more generally.

For example, Trudy Patterson (sixty, white, working poor/impoverished), who was described in Chapter 3 as having a rather functional approach to food, commented that she was "not big on cooking." Viewing food as a necessity, she preferred easy dishes. With her limited resources, her diet was admittedly narrow, and she did not eat out much. Trudy's aversion to vegetarian eating – explicitly expressed in a response to a photo of hummus and falafel – seemed to draw on a cultural repertoire that privileged the familiar meat-and-potatoes menu (see Chapter 7 for Trudy's case study). She linked vegetarianism with unfamiliar eating, employing a tentative response to cosmopolitanism, as detailed in Chapter 3:

No, I wouldn't eat that [hummus and falafel]. It's just unappealing to me, and I don't like trying different foods really. That's just unappealing. I wouldn't know what was in it, how it tasted, so I'd be kind of turned off of it. Vegetarians would be more into that sort of stuff, and I don't plan to be a vegetarian. Because I like meat.

Though she had vegetarian friends, Trudy had no idea of what food to serve them or where to take them to eat.

Todd Roberts (sixteen, white, working poor/impoverished) expressed a similar lack of interest in and connection to vegetarianism. He had "never thought about being a vegetarian before" and believed that it was an unhealthy choice. Todd's forty-nine-year-old mother, Toni, said she was "not an adventurous eater" and characterized a proper evening meal as featuring meat, potatoes, and vegetables:

> Supper's a big thing. We'll have pork chops; we'll have corn or potatoes, things that go together. A certain kind of main dish and a certain kind of vegetable go together. We like our meat! We like our potatoes! Growing up, this is what we ate. My mom didn't have time to, you know, make special dinners for all of us. It just didn't happen.

Toni's repertoire regarding food and proper eating appears to have been learned in her family of origin, where children ate what they were served and were not catered to with special meals.

In combination with the lack of material resources that would enable experimentation with food, this kind of cultural repertoire indicates why families with differing economic and cultural capital may respond differently to a teen's vegetarianism. When priorities centre on family patterns, familiarity, and a traditional approach to healthy eating, adoption of vegetarianism could be highly disruptive. Conversely, the middle-class parents who supported children's vegetarianism had access to material resources, a culinary repertoire that might already include meatless dishes, an experimental approach to food, the ability to inform themselves, and the belief that vegetarianism was a healthy option.

Vegetarian Teens and the Good Parent

Particular class-based discourses (Foucault 1979, 1980) could enable individuals to constitute themselves as good parents through their responses to teen vegetarianism (see Chapter 1 for a discussion of good mothering and healthy eating). Supportive parents appeared to draw on a middle-class parenting discourse that is intensely child-centred, promoting children's rights to make autonomous decisions (see Bassett, Chapman, and Beagan 2008). In supporting their teen's vegetarianism, they displayed their version of good parenting. In contrast, those who resisted were also engaging in good parenting; it was simply a different version.

As mentioned above, all the resistant parents were low income and working class or working poor/impoverished. The fact that some low-income families were supportive, however, suggests that opposition was not solely a product of limited material resources, but also incorporated cultural repertoires concerning eating and parenting. Resistant parents did not purchase vegetarian foods or prepare meatless options. Some pressured their children to eat meat during family meals (see Roth 2005; Merriman 2010). Not surprisingly, the teens typically returned to meat eating after a few days or months. These families talked about arguments and described the teens' attempts to become vegetarian as conflictual.

Most parents who opposed teen vegetarianism did so on the basis of health, invoking the "traditional" healthy eating discourse, which emphasizes that meals should consist of meat and vegetables. As we suggested in Chapter 1, this discourse circulates through personal experience and family teachings. People refer to the way in which their parents and grandparents ate – it was good enough for them, so it's good enough now. Resistant parents who subscribed to this discourse believed that vegetarianism translated to insufficient nutrition. Fearing negative health consequences for their children, they sometimes pressured them to revert to meat eating. Kelsey Kidston (forty-two, white, working poor/impoverished) recalled nutrition-related discussions with her thirteen-year-old daughter, Kaleigh: "She tried to go on that vegetarian kick a little while ago. We talked about it first, and she was showing interest in it. And I said, 'Well, you're gonna have to eat beans and stuff for protein. And peanut butter.' And she's, like, 'No, I don't like that.' And I said, 'Well, you're not gonna be a vegetarian.'" In this case, Kaleigh's reluctance to eat alternative sources of protein closed the door on vegetarianism – for both mother and daughter. Good parenting here is enacted through protecting health.

Parents sometimes repelled teen vegetarianism because they saw it as a "hard" dietary lifestyle, whereas meat-based diets were perceived as "easy." They found that shopping and cooking for vegetarian meals was difficult and time consuming, as was offering meatless options such as veggie dogs or the "chicken" slices mentioned by Trish Rendell above. Clearly, if particular culinary or cultural repertoires facilitate support for vegetarianism, parents whose repertoires differ will find support to be far more challenging and time consuming. When material resources are limited – including the time for extra shopping or cooking – and the necessary skills and experimentation are not already in place, accommodating teen vegetarianism will be far more difficult.

For some parents, supporting teen vegetarianism contradicted their understandings of the best approach to raising children. The good parenting discourses that predominate in middle-class Western milieus may not be as enthusiastically endorsed by working-class families and migrants (Lareau 2002, 2011; Thorsted and Anving 2010). In the working class, and especially in families on income assistance, heightened vulnerability to state surveillance (through schools, health professionals, and social workers) may increase the need to portray themselves as "good parents" through careful control of their children (Gilliom 2001) and adherence to traditionally accepted approaches to feeding the family. The child-centred parenting of middle-class circles (Bassett, Chapman, and Beagan 2008) may be perceived as overly indulgent and accommodating.

In the case study above, Tenzing Pasang converted to vegetarianism for religious-ethical reasons but returned to meat after a few months. Although his mother, Tara, was familiar with vegetarianism because she was a Tibetan Buddhist (it was thus within her cultural repertoire), she resisted buying or preparing special meatless foods for Tenzing. As he remarked,

> I tried to be a vegetarian for, like, two or three months, and it didn't quite work out so well because me and my mom kind of had arguments once in a while. I think it's hard for her to make

two separate kinds of food just for me. It's hard to make things without meat that the whole family will eat. And I can't make pasta or ravioli if I don't have them, if I don't have the ingredients ... which my mom decides.

Accommodating Tenzing's vegetarian efforts was challenging for Tara because it created extra work for her, but perhaps she also felt that indulging individual preferences benefitted neither the child nor the family.

Parents who supported teen vegetarianism sometimes worried about its healthfulness, an anxiety that could result in extra measures to manage their children's diets. Some consulted with nutrition experts and strove to empower the teens themselves with knowledge about food and cooking. For example, Katrina Kellough (forty-six, white, working poor/impoverished) had once been a community outreach worker who educated others about healthy eating and thus had some work-related food education. When her daughter decided to become a vegetarian, Katrina took her to consult with medical experts – a family doctor and a nutritionist – to ensure that her dietary needs were being met. In addition, she made considerable efforts to source affordable vegetarian products to ensure that her daughter had sufficient protein. Katrina spoke about the work entailed in tracking down the vegetarian burger that her daughter liked and that she herself could afford:

> There's certain places, not in Kingston, you can really get her kinds of foods much, much cheaper. There's one in Napanee that's a country food market, and I just became aware of one in Belleville and basically, whatever you call, her kind of hamburger, her kind of chicken breast, chicken fingers, everything. All vegetarian, which she really likes. You can mostly only find them in Loblaw's here, and the price is huge ... So, we really buy lots of those when we go to those places and put it in the freezer for her. So we give her variety.

Other parents also went to great lengths to support their children's vegetarianism – which clearly required ample time, if not material resources. Tammy Raikatuji (forty-seven, Japanese Canadian, lower middle class) devoted tremendous effort to providing a wide range of high-end vegetarian foods for her fifteen-year-old daughter Tracey, despite the family's low income:

> I have gone to the nth degree to buy – oh, that's where I would indulge in is vegetarian. I absolutely indulge in vegetarian food for my daughter. I probably spend eight or nine dollars on vegetarian marshmallows that I tracked down for, like, a month ... I buy, like, all the veg, meat substitutes. Or things that might be a novelty in that area. A lot of soy products. I would buy a lot of things that are really specific to her that we could eat. I don't know how many types of different kinds of beans – organics and otherwise – that I have stocked.

Tammy's prioritization of serving a panoply of vegetarian and organic foods speaks to an increasingly common ideal of upper-middle-class parenting, in which a "good mother" provides healthy food but also seeks to raise a "pure," "organic child," protected from chemicals, pesticides, and harmful additives (Cairns, Johnston, and MacKendrick 2013). Tammy's evident pride in her support for Tracey's vegetarianism suggests that she was presenting herself as a good mother via a parenting style that endorsed children's autonomous choices.

In keeping with this middle-class discourse, supportive parents took their children's beliefs and preferences very seriously. For example, Kristal Chirnian (forty-two, white, upper middle class) described her response when her daughter Kallie (fifteen) decided to become vegetarian:

> I remember it well because it was a very stressful time in my life, and it was an issue at first. But then the parenting bit kicked in, and I recentred and obviously I am going to respect what she wants, and there is nothing wrong with a vegetarian diet. In fact, it's probably been a wonderful impact overall. Kallie's dietary needs and wants directed how we all sit down and eat the same food now.

Similarly, Brenda Voisey (forty-nine, Irish Canadian, working poor/ impoverished) strongly supported her daughter's decision to be a vegetarian, explaining that she would not serve meat to vegetarian guests, which would be insulting, so she accorded the same respect to her daughter's choices. Like Kristal, Brenda noted that her daughter's vegetarianism had positively influenced her own eating style. Whereas resistant parents experienced their children's vegetarianism as challenging and difficult to implement, supportive parents (primarily mothers) seemed to incorporate it thoroughly and effortlessly. The easiness of the transition could be a rewriting of history, however, as it had occurred several years before for most families. Nevertheless, themes of struggle and conflict were not at the forefront of these recollections, and parents spoke about their desire to oblige children's preferences in very positive terms.

THE IMPACT OF TEEN VEGETARIANISM

Although some studies suggest that family reactions to teen vegetarianism are largely negative (see, for example, Roth 2005), most parents in our study neither resisted it nor attempted to maintain meat-eating traditions in the family. Indeed, most families supported teen vegetarianism in a variety of ways. The highest degree of this occurred in six families who moved toward eating more vegetarian food themselves: two converted to vegetarianism after the teenager did, and four increased their overall consumption of meatless food. In these families, only two parents had previously been vegetarian. Thus, behavioural influence in a family can be multidirectional – in this case, a change in teen eating modified the family eating style.

In some instances, familial changes were made to respect the preference of the teen, as in the case of Brenda Voisey (above), who felt that serving meat to a vegetarian was inappropriate and disrespectful. However, accommodations were sometimes more pragmatically motivated, seeking to make life easier for the mother, who was usually the primary cook and who preferred not to make two meals. In keeping with Canadian trends (Beagan et al. 2008), foodwork in our 105 study families was done mostly by mothers, including meal preparation and shopping. When men participated, it was usually in exceptional circumstances (as when the father was retired, had non-standard employment hours, or contributed in circumscribed ways such as doing all the barbecuing). Thus, mothers who cooked the same vegetarian meal for every family member could reduce their labour.

Initially, parents often cooked two separate meals to accommodate a teen vegetarian but then realized that serving one vegetarian meal for everyone would be easier. Aaron Adams (fourteen, Latvian Scottish Canadian, upper middle class) recalled that his mother had cooked separate meals until it became "too difficult." His mother, Annette, eventually stopped wanting meat:

> Aaron has been a vegetarian much longer than me. He became a vegetarian for principle reasons, and I became a vegetarian because I stopped craving meat. So for many years I was cooking two dishes. So I was cooking the pasta and then the sauce. And I'd be cooking the meat separately. I would serve him the pasta and the sauce, and then I'd put the meat on mine. So, yeah, I would do two different meals. So I was eating meats ... for quite a while after he became vegetarian, and then I just stopped craving it.

Similarly, Trish Rendell stated that everyone in her family "just got used to not having meat" in meals. In these situations, reduced meat consumption gradually became more habitual in the family.

Some mothers said that having a vegetarian child led to dietary changes that they appreciated and even enjoyed. As a result of altering their habits, they experienced pleasure and a sense of satisfaction in trying new foods. They framed their children's vegetarianism as an accomplishment in which they themselves took pride. Kristal Chirnian (forty-two, white, upper middle class) admired her daughter Kallie's decision to be a vegetarian and valued its healthy impact on her family:

> If I were to say, if someone was doing a parenting study and they were to say, what makes you proud? It makes me proud if my kids eat different things! I look at what we eat at dinner, when we eat together, we eat really well. I think it's healthy food, it's primarily low fat but always has protein. I think we eat pretty well now. But I think for Kallie, her dietary needs and wants directed that. Because as I came away from eating so much meat and eating more rounded food – like, when I wasn't afraid to eat a bean any more – it was good!

Other supportive mothers felt that their children's vegetarianism had rejuvenated their own interest in cooking. For some, the challenge of preparing meatless dishes had remedied their lack of confidence in their cooking skills. Brenda Voisey (forty-nine, Irish Canadian, working poor/impoverished) thought that making vegetarian meals involved "higher-level cooking skills" because it required more consciousness about where food came from. She had tried a variety of meat substitutes and discovered that she enjoyed them more than her daughter Brogan did.

Several other supportive parents who found themselves enjoying vegetarian food mentioned the unexpected side effects of feeling healthier and experiencing desired weight loss. Nuala Haldane (forty, white, working class) not only acquired new cooking skills, but also made new connections at work when she swapped recipes with colleagues who were interested in healthy eating and cooking, a network that included administrative staff and health professionals:

> I've made sesame noodles and orange raisin couscous salad. It was so good the girl at work took it from me. She said, "That looks some good!" I'm like, "It is good." See, I've been trying to get these vegetarian foods [online]. One of the doctors made this salad at work, so then I said I'll make it for my daughter. So I'm trying to, you know, adapt.

Nuala reported that by eating more vegetarian food with her daughter, she had also lost a significant amount of weight.

As a final point – and something of a counterpoint – though our data show that children could influence parents to eat vegetarian, the opposite occurred in three families, where teens convinced vegetarian parents to reintroduce meat into their diets. In all three instances, this change accommodated the wishes of teenage sons. Though the numbers are too small to indicate clear patterns, this seems to suggest a particular gender effect, in keeping with our comments in Chapter 1 – that meat eating is masculine. Thus, denying meat to adolescent boys may pose particular challenges. In these three families, the mothers did most of the foodwork, and all started to eat meat themselves once they were cooking it for male family members, to reduce the burden of making separate meals. Although the outcome in these families differed from instances where children prompted their parents to pursue vegetarian diets, the point remains that family eating may change in response to the food preferences of teens.

CONCLUSION

Our study participants demonstrated that the family reaction to teen vegetarianism depended on both material resources and cultural repertoire, one of which is vegetarianism itself. Access to this repertoire was shaped by cultural and economic capital. Supportive parents were predominantly middle class or working class or working poor who had experienced downward mobility. Some had been vegetarian themselves and saw it as a healthy option. Their support seemed to overlap with other aspects of middle-class consumption and perhaps also intersected with a parenting style that respected children's independence (Lareau 2002). Many of these parents were readily able to incorporate teen diet preferences, even when the change was costly, inconvenient, and labour-intensive. Families that converted to vegetarianism did so because they saw it as healthy and because it eliminated the work of preparing two separate meals. By contrast, all resistant parents were low-income members of the working class. Their opposition may have arisen from their limited material resources, a cultural repertoire that saw meat as integral to healthy eating, and a parenting mode that emphasized respect for authority (Lareau 2002, 2011; Thorsted and Anving 2010).

5

body image

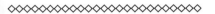

The Keating Family

THE KEATINGS ARE a white, working-class family who live on the outskirts of Kingston, Ontario. Katherine Keating (forty-three) is a single parent of Keri (fourteen) and Keegan (twenty), both of whom live at home. Katherine, who works as an administrative assistant at a local hospital, has an annual income of about $50,000 – well below the median family income for Kingston. The Keatings live on one side of a duplex, and Katherine's father, Keith Kafton, lives on the other side. There is a great deal of movement between the two households, particularly in relation to food. Katherine commonly cooks supper for her father, and Keegan and Keri often raid their grandfather's fridge for snacks.

There is significant tension in the household with regard to body weight and body image. Katherine is concerned about her own weight as well as that of her daughter, Keri, and is dissatisfied with the family's eating habits. She describes their diet as "normal," "plain," and "meat and potatoes." Although meals are often prepared from scratch, they also include some "really nasty foods" in which the family "indulges." Katherine herself is fond of chips and describes Keri and Keegan as "pop-aholics" who like sweets. Katherine's father, Keith, eats prepared foods such as canned pasta.

Disturbed about her recent weight gain, Katherine has begun deleting some starches and phasing out potatoes from family meals:

> I'm so sedentary all winter. I'll sit on that couch – I mean, once the house-work's done, that's it, that's where I sit. And I've said for years now, "I'm moving out of this house. That's it, I'm moving into the city." 'Cause I can get an apartment, and then I'll be walking the streets. I'll do my shopping, I'll get my exercise. Here, once I'm home and it's winter ... I'm on the couch, eating my chips. And I have gained about fifteen pounds this winter.

Katherine's father tends to monitor her weight, at one point saying to her, "Dear, you've got to do something about your weight!" Though she has mis-givings about the amount of sugar that her children consume, because of the "diabetes concern," she is most worried about Keri. She describes her son Keegan as "a rake" and her daughter as "quite overweight."

Despite Katherine's anxiety about Keri's weight, she cannot get their family doctor to take the issue seriously. She is also frustrated that her father, Keith, supplies Keri with snacks such as Pop-Tarts and Toaster Strudels: "That's more than likely what Keri's doing over there [at Keith's], is getting a snack. And that's another issue we constantly deal with, Dad and I, is the back and forth. When I say, 'No, you're done,' and if I go to bed early, she's right over there, eating."

Though Katherine describes Keri as "very aware of her weight issue" and "constantly making an effort to get things under control and change the way she eats," Keri herself seems quite undisturbed about the subject. She doesn't eat at McDonald's, as much to shun food preservatives as to avoid potential weight gain. When asked if she or her peers dieted and were con-cerned about body image, she said no. Despite her mother's worries, she does not diet for weight loss: "I'm allowed to have whatever. But certain things my mom's like, 'Well, you shouldn't be eating that at this time,' be-cause it's not healthy. But I just really grab whatever there is, if I'm really hungry."

Whereas Katherine is alarmed about Keri's weight and often associates this anxiety with her own weight-loss projects, Keri resists her mother's problematization of her body and insists on her own set of rules about healthy eating and body size.

· · · *The Esani Family*

THE ESANIS ARE an upper-middle-class South Asian Canadian family who live in Edmonton. They have been in Alberta for six years, having emigrated from Pakistan. The mother of the family, Adeela (forty-one), is a full-time social worker and also does all the cooking for her sons Aarya (twenty) and Arjan (fourteen), and daughter Amara (eighteen). Due to the demands of his job, Adeela's husband, Abdul, spends most of his time in a nearby city and is home for only a few days each month. Adeela makes all his food, freezing dishes throughout the month for him to take back with him. Their annual income is about $90,000, well above the median for Edmonton.

Food is a contentious topic among the Esanis. As Adeela notes, "Most of the fights in our household are around food." This is particularly the case for Adeela and her son Aarya, who is a student at the local university. She always cooks South Asian dishes such as biryani and takes great pride in her ability to prepare healthy Pakistani food from scratch; she is dismayed by Aarya's consumption of Western food at campus eateries and believes that it is responsible for what she describes as his "obesity":

> When I come home, my son will phone from campus, "What did you cook today?" And I'll say this. He goes, "Oh, I don't like this, I'm eating out." And then the tension starts, eh? "But I cooked it from scratch, this is fresh." "But I don't like it, so I'm eating out." And I say, "Oh, you're gaining so much weight, you're always eating out." So the tension starts.

Concerned about Aarya's weight, Adeela is discouraged by the fact that he seems to do nothing about it. When asked if she had mentioned this to him, she replied,

> So many times! A hundred, two hundred times. He has a gym membership, he doesn't go there. He's lazy ... And he thinks that he's still young, and young people don't get sick. "Who cares, if I'm forty, then I'll get sick at that point." He doesn't care. Just laziness and carelessness and a teenage

attitude ... Everybody has talked to him ... My sisters, my brothers, my sisters-in-law – everybody ... He didn't care. What else can we do? He went to the doctor, his cholesterol is not that bad, actually, but he is obese.

Aarya himself worries about neither his weight, body image, nor health: "I don't feel much of that. I mean, I want to be healthy and stuff, but I don't see it as too extreme." He acknowledges eating out quite often during school days but does try to choose healthy menu items and disagrees with his mother that eating out is necessarily unhealthy: "When I get something, I don't get fries on the side, I get a salad, just to keep it balanced, I guess. We usually keep away from the fried food. I know I should *[laughs]*. I guess, just proportions – sometimes even home foods are not healthy."

Aarya insists that homemade Pakistani food is not necessarily healthy: "It's oily ... It's not all healthy for sure. Only if you're eating, like, lentils or something, right? That would be different. But here, it's, like, chicken curry or the meatballs are, like, beef and oil, I don't know. Or if you're eating, like, vegetable, then it's different. But what we eat, it's not really healthy." His mother strongly disagrees, pointing out that her younger son, who eats at home, is much slimmer.

In this conflict, Aarya's sister, Amara, aligns with her mother. She argues that eating non-Western food at home is healthier because it promotes weight loss: "I know what's in it ... and I can portion my food." She takes on some surveillance of her brothers: "They eat a lot of junk food. I try to tell them not to eat the junk food, but they don't care *[laughs]*." She herself does not eat "junk food" and in fact tries to eat very little:

I'm not really exactly calorie counting but just if I know that I ate really heavy during lunch, I probably would just not eat dinner, just make myself milk and cereal or just milk and toast. I usually don't even eat dinner. I usually try to avoid it, but my mom just gets on my back and she's like, "Why aren't you eating? You're supposed to be eating," you know? But I try to avoid it.

Interestingly, Adeela expresses no concern about this.

Amara also limits her snacking to foods that are "either a hundred or ninety calories" and exercises at the gym for at least an hour every day. She sees her restricted diet as an important part of being a "health person":

I'm a big, big health person, so usually, like, my snacks or something, if I take it to school, it'll be, like, this granola bar and then all this hundred-calorie stuff ... Because I mean two cookies are like two hundred calories! That's just too much, you know? And then especially because I work out, I look at how much time it takes me to burn off those two hundred calories, so, like, oh my God, if I'm eating just one cookie, it's like a half an hour gone right there.

Amara attributes her restricted diet and intense exercise regime to the pressures that girls face to be thin, "like models that are ten times smaller than you," and also to peers who "like to stay skinny." At one point in her life, they had "totally put [her] down" for being "super fat." Amara relates, "In Grade nine, I felt they were really watching me ... For sure, my friends played a part."

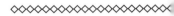

IN THE ESANI family, the gender differences in weight maintenance regimes are evident. Both Aarya and Amara are subject to scrutiny, but whereas Aarya is able to resist it, Amara is not, due in part to wider standards regarding the female body. However, Adeela's anxieties concerning Aarya's "obesity" suggest that ideals of thinness may be increasingly directed at boys and men, often via the language of "health" and "healthy eating."

As demonstrated by the Keatings and the Esanis, body image was important to many participants in our study, even if they often framed it as being about "health." For the most part, these concerns focused on "excess" body fat and overweight. Some interviewees were on commercial diets to lose weight or had been in the past. Many restricted food informally. Most, as described in Chapter 1, simply attempted to "eat healthy," which is often directly related to weight control.

As feminist literature reveals, weight control issues are not gender-neutral. In our sample, they were most commonly discussed by women and girls, but men and boys also expressed an interest in the topic. Whereas this was often filtered through the more acceptable health discourse, boys in particular raised concerns about extra body fat, inches, and pounds in ways that were reminiscent of traditionally feminine concerns.

THEORETICAL FRAMING

Body image issues as they apply to women and girls have been thoroughly discussed by many feminist scholars (see, for example, Chernin 1985; Wolf 1992; Bordo 1993). In the main, feminist literature focuses on gendering the experience of disordered eating such as anorexia and bulimia, but it also examines more prosaic behaviours such as dieting, the close monitoring of weight, and excessive exercise (Rice 2007). These are mostly undertaken by women and girls who strive toward a slim ideal that is neither attainable nor healthy for most people.

Feminist scholars have long argued that body image is disproportionately a feminine issue, rooted in patriarchal social systems that privilege men and subordinate women. Some suggest that the pressure to diet springs from a not-so-hidden belief that a "good woman" must take up as little space as possible (see Chernin 1985). The slim ideal is seen as distracting women's attentions and energies from more important endeavours (Wolf 1992). Inspired by psychoanalysis, some scholars suggest that body fat itself is intrinsically feminine because it is necessary to the female reproductive process (Kent 2001; McPhail 2009). Thus, fat can be seen as a feminine entity that must be expunged or at least tightly controlled to eliminate the socially subordinated status that it symbolizes. Other scholars maintain that when mind and body are understood as separate, as in Cartesian dualism (see Bordo 1993; Bartky 1997; Rice 2007), women are conflated with the body and men with the seemingly higher realm of cognition and the mind (Grosz 1994). In turn, women are subject to and subjects of a variety of techniques to control the body, such as weight loss and maintenance, which are designed to contain and constrain – but also produce – their embodiment.

As we pointed out in Chapter 1, dominant discourses discipline people and govern their actions in part through making them responsible for behaving as good citizens, good men, and good women (Foucault 1979, 1980). Self-monitoring is integral to this process. Weight-loss techniques can be understood as just this kind of "discipline"

(Bartky 1997). Diet and exercise are important disciplinary techniques through which women may create and articulate their identities, by engaging in practices that are perceived as feminine and by the resultant production of feminized bodies. Thus, engagement in the "war on fat" (Rice 2007) can be seen as helping to lay the groundwork for women's very sense of themselves not only as women, but as subjects or *selves*. At the same time, self-monitoring and the techniques of weight loss define the body as an object to be scrutinized and controlled. Women are therefore in the precarious position of constructing their sense of self as an object for the enjoyment of others (Young 2005) – pieces of flesh to be looked at, weighed, measured, and reduced.

Such conflation of femininity with the disciplined removal of fat has recently come into question, particularly with the discursive emergence of a so-called obesity epidemic. The explosion of concern about obesity in health, academic, and public circles has not been directed exclusively at women (Biltekoff 2013). Indeed, as some national statistics show higher rates of obesity in men than in women (Public Health Agency of Canada and the Canadian Institute for Health Information 2011), women's practices of diet and exercise have been hailed as healthy and enviable (Kirkey 2008). Popular TV shows that feature weight loss and magazines such as *Men's Health* profile men's slim-down techniques through restrictive diets and exercise. It seems that men are increasingly subject to disciplinary regimes of weight maintenance and that they, too, must now be slim to be conform with ideal masculinity (Gilman 2004; Bell and McNaughton 2007; Monaghan 2008; McPhail 2009; Norman 2011, 2013). In large part, this has arisen from the expansive obesity discourse and the move from weight loss for appearance to the seemingly common sense equation of weight loss with health (Norman 2011). This new emphasis has encouraged men to engage in weight maintenance regimes "for health" while still portraying themselves as masculine because they are not dieting for appearance.

Despite these increasing pressures on men, it is important to note that body image remains a highly gendered issue, in that men and women do not experience weight-loss directives in the same ways or to the same degree. As Norman (2011, 433) argues, "The pressures men experience should not lead one to conclude that men are equal victims of the 'beauty myth.'" Thinness remains a central characteristic of femininity – to be a "good" woman, one must be thin or at least attempting to be so, whereas men can be largely unconcerned with weight and still remain "real" men. In our study, this difference was evident in the degrees to which Amara and Aarya Esani could resist or submit to pressures to diet. Certainly, Amara felt pressures outside the home that were not experienced by her brother, and the attitudes of her girlfriends regarding her weight speak to the gendered ways in which expectations are enforced. However, though weight loss remains paramount to women and girls, it is imperative to trace the ways in which body image is increasingly of interest to men and boys (Beausoleil and Ward 2010).

PARTICIPANTS, PLACES, AND APPROACH TO ANALYSIS

This chapter uses data from Alberta and eastern Ontario, concentrating on interviews with eleven families in Edmonton and ten in Athabasca County, Alberta, plus thirteen families in Kingston and nine in Prince Edward County. The sample included forty-three women, five men, thirty-two girls, and twenty-three boys.

WOMEN, GIRLS, AND BODY IMAGE

As we noted in Chapter 1, most women and girls in British Columbia and Nova Scotia expressed some dissatisfaction with their weight or bodies, generally connecting this to discourses of health and healthy eating. Alberta and eastern Ontario yielded similar results, with no obvious differences between these two sites. For example, Karla Cleveland (forty-two, white, upper middle class) had recently lost forty pounds through "cutting out the crap and ramping up some exercise." Explaining her motives, she noted that she "just [wanted] to try and have a bit better health." Demonstrating a high degree of awareness regarding medical measures for body size and shape, Anezka Embler (sixteen, white, upper middle class) stated, "I've always been fiftieth percentile for height and ninetieth for weight since I was very young." Her doctor had recently warned her that she was becoming too heavy and suggested she change her diet to what she described as "healthier."

[The doctor] told my mom she should think of healthier alternatives for all the family, because it would be hard for me all by
myself to make this change. And my mom has tried to make
healthier meals – a lot less pasta, whole grain things, vegetables
… And I've been trying to keep up my end of the deal. I think my
doctor should be happy.

For many, the very definition of health itself was tied to weight, thus
echoing mainstream discourses of health promotion. When asked to
describe healthy eating, for instance, Alison Ahenakew (forty-eight,
Cree, working poor/impoverished) replied,

The word "healthy eating" would mean to me finding a balance
between nutrition and your physical fitness, I guess. Finding
food that you can eat, that you like, that is good for you as far
as nutrition, but that can also be balanced by a certain degree of
exercise or physical activity that kind of balances the two of
them, so you're not too – either under- or overweight.

Similarly, Ashley Elliott (sixteen, white, working class) described the
disparate eating styles in her divorced parents' homes: she felt unhealthy at her father's house because she ate more treats, whereas
she felt healthy at her mother's because of its more health-conscious
environment. Ashley linked health and healthy eating directly to
weight: "I wouldn't want to eat completely at my dad's house, because
I would eventually feel fat, like, health-wise."

To achieve what they felt were "healthy" weights, women and girls
in Alberta and eastern Ontario participated in disciplinary techniques,
as mentioned in the feminist literature on body image. Some were on
commercial diets, some restricted their food intake, and others followed exercise programs designed to control weight. Alina Eliszewski
(fifty-two, white, upper middle class) had joined Weight Watchers "a
couple of years ago" and lost twenty-five pounds. She said that she
"need[ed] to get back to it" because she had recently "put on ten." In
explaining her interest in the Weight Watchers diet, Alina referred to
healthy eating: "So you count points, and different kinds of food have
different points. And if you want to lose weight, you're allowed up to a
certain number of points in a day … So, you know, it's healthy for

everybody to eat like that." By our second interview, Alina had re-enrolled in Weight Watchers. Her seveneen-year-old daughter, Aureli, had also lost "a bunch of weight" over the last year due to a change in diet, "eating less stuff and eating more reasonable food like more whole grains." Although Aureli was not in Weight Watchers, she did eat the Weight Watchers food that her mother had in the house.

Like Amara Esani, Aliya Edo-Khel (thirty-seven, Pakistani, upper middle class) tried to control her weight through diet restriction and exercise, though she found exercising difficult:

> I don't want to get fat or put too much weight on. I was exercis-ing. When I was back home [in Pakistan], I was doing exercise a lot, and I would walk every day for forty-five minutes there. But when I came here, like, the weather [in Edmonton] is totally dif-ferent here. You can't go outside every day for a walk, so I try to go to [local gym] for some time, but then I quit because I didn't have much time. So now I'm trying to control my diet ... I try not to eat too much rice. And naan too. Because the main reason you put on weight is if you eat too much naan.

Corroborating the feminist literature on body image, women and girls in our study often said, both directly and indirectly, that their weight management measures were integral to their identities. For Ashley Elliott (sixteen, white, working class) a recent weight gain left her feeling not quite herself, which she framed in terms of health: "I'm fine with the weight I am if I felt healthy, but I feel like I'm under a cloud most of the time." Kristal Chirnian (forty-two, white, upper middle class) similarly described a sense of discomfort with a recent weight gain and reminisced about a time when she felt better and "firmer" – even as she chastised herself for connecting self-worth to her physical appearance:

> When I say, like, a healthy weight for me, 130, 135 [pounds], is like, that standard size ten, just comfortable. Not skinny by any stretch of the imagination, but just – and fit feeling. Meaning firmer feeling than looser feeling, so I know that I am exercising – is where I feel most comfortable. The only way I have ever been able to maintain that in my whole adult life was to completely go

off the carbohydrates, and I lived on no more than twenty grams of carbohydrate a day for four years, maintained a 120 to 130 range in my weight and honestly I don't think I ever felt better. I felt really physically good, and I felt good because I felt like I looked good. I'm rolling my eyes, because it's so vain, but it's the truth.

This distancing from feminine beauty ideals, as expressed in Kristal's remark about the vanity of wanting to be thin, was common among women and girls in the study. That is, even as fat avoidance, weight-loss regimes, and the desire for slimness were prevalent, many participants also named, resented, and sometimes resisted the pressure to obtain the "ideal" body.

Alison Ahenakew (forty-eight, Cree, working poor/impoverished) noted this social pressure:

> It seems to be that most women are not comfortable with their weight. Either they're too heavy or too light or too this or too that. It seems to me, of the two sexes, women are the most … like, even in the commercials you see on TV, the diet programs and stuff are aimed at the women more than the men.

Thus, Alison identified the sexism of dieting culture, adeptly capturing a feminist critique of the media emphasis on feminine slenderness.

Indeed, this critique seemed to be common sense for many women and girls, who recognized the gender inequity of the weight-loss edicts. However, they responded to this imbalance in differing ways. Some avoided food restriction. For example, when asked whether weight considerations influenced her food choice, Kristi Keller (thirty-nine, white, working poor/impoverished) replied, "I think for women, yeah. For sure there is. For me personally, no. There hasn't. I eat when I'm hungry; I eat whatever I want." More commonly, though participants were aware of the pressure to diet, they nonetheless took it up. April Enman (forty-four, white, working poor/impoverished) described herself as "definitely" concerned about her weight and as attempting to decrease it by controlling her food intake. Yet she was also frustrated with "unhealthy" Western definitions of beauty, comparing them to those of Pakistan, her husband's country of origin:

Definitely they did have concerns about body image and it was important, but it was not at all like – it was healthy to me, healthier, like, there wasn't overly thin people at all. I mean, they definitely wanted to have nice figures, but it wasn't that pressure put on women. It was less advertising and everything, right? The girls that were portrayed as pretty would probably be considered overweight here.

Girls also expressed both an awareness of and resistance to dominant beauty ideals, which were often perpetuated by their mothers. In the case studies above, Keri Keating and Amara Esani exemplify two ways in which girls responded to the anti-fat discourses voiced by their mothers. Keri avoided McDonald's due to the anti-obesity discourse, yet her peer group resisted pressures to diet, and she herself did not share her mother's focus on weight loss. Amara critiqued the fact that girls are pressured to look like "models that are ten times smaller than you." For her, however, critique of the discourse did not translate into resistance. She strictly controlled both her diet and her weight in an approach that aligned with her mother's concerns about weight and the equation of thinness with health.

Other girls interacted in differing ways with social, peer, and parental interpretations of beauty ideals. Aureli Eliszewski (seventeen, white, upper middle class) mentioned both the pressure to diet and the difficulty of resisting: "You know, teenage girls are really concerned with [body image]. My group of friends doesn't care about that as much, but we still kind of pay attention to it because you have to. We're inundated with that stuff all of the time. But it's less of an issue for my group of friends than for somebody else."

Though she added that Hollywood images of women are unrealistic, Aureli had also recently lost weight, sharing her mother's concerns with weight loss and weight maintenance (and her Weight Watchers food). Sisters Atifa and Azra Edo-Khel (fourteen and thirteen, Pakistani and Euro-Canadian, upper middle class) reported that their mother, who was "very conscious" about her own weight, had attempted to regulate their weight since moving to Edmonton from Pakistan: "If our mom sees us taking this big serving of fries, like, really big, then she's, like, 'That's too much. You're going to gain weight.' Things like that." Asked if body image was a common topic in their circle, Atifa replied, "No, not really. They talk about it in the house, because my mom's like 'You have to lose weight' ... In the house my mom was telling [Anwar] to gain weight and telling me to lose weight. But at school no one really talks about it."

In contrast to some others, Kaleigh Kidston (thirteen, white, working poor/impoverished) apparently did not reject dominant body image discourses, having recently incorporated them into her everyday food practices. She related a weight loss of forty pounds following a visit to her extended family:

> My grandma and my aunt and my grandpa, and my aunts, they're all kind of on the heavier side, and so I do not want to be like that. So I decided to lose weight. I lost almost forty pounds ... I ate *way* less than I used to ... And I've started to eat whole wheat ... I stopped eating French fries. I don't really eat much junk food.

Although Kaleigh's mother, Kelsey (forty-two), was proud of her weight loss, she worried about what she called "the whole 'I don't want to be fat' thing" in that Kaleigh wasn't getting "enough food ... enough nutrition." This sometimes caused conflict, as Kelsey tried to convince Kaleigh to eat breakfast or lunch by threatening to "limit her time on the computer."

Whereas Kaleigh acted on the body image discourse despite (conflicted) opposition from her mother, Karol Karsten (twelve, white, working class) recognized the ways in which her peers implemented it, though she herself did not. She expressed guilt about her resistance:

> I think that I eat a lot more than them [my friends]. 'Cause you look in their lunch pails, and some days they don't even bring something sugary. It's all fruit, vegetables − like, the junkiest things some of my friends bring is pretzels. And then I look in my lunch pail, and sometimes I'll have a Kool-Aid Jammer and a honey bun. So, it's kind of awkward 'cause you're just sitting there eating something junky. And if they bring chips, it's, like ... the healthiest ones. So I kind of feel bad, 'cause they're all so thin and healthy ... And I'm just, I swim and eat food.

Even though Karol fended off the pressure to diet, she nonetheless engaged in self-surveillance and monitoring the food intake of others.

Like women, the girls in the study responded in complicated ways to the body image discourse, either rejecting it (with or without guilt), practising it but remaining critical, or taking it up without apparent reservations. In many cases, their responses to beauty ideals were connected to those of their peers and mothers. In turn, like most Canadians, women regarded weight loss and maintenance as healthy, and were thus enacting "good" mothering when they urged their daughters to achieve it (see Chapter 1).

This maternal caretaking of weight also shows the significant role that mothers may play in girls' relationship to beauty ideals. In addition, our data demonstrate that, bombarded as they are by medical and popular rhetoric about childhood and adolescent obesity, mothers are pushed to raise healthy children who have no weight "problems" – a reality that is beginning to influence their interactions with their sons.

MASCULINITY AND BODY WEIGHT DISCOURSES
As noted in Chapter 1, few men in British Columbia and Nova Scotia discussed weight loss or weight maintenance regimens. Although there were fewer men in our sample, even those who did participate apparently regarded weight loss as a feminine domain. Those who did diet tended to recuperate the masculinity lost through dieting in other ways, a process of "masculinity insurance" (Anderson 2002; see also Lyons 2009). Similarly, very few men in Alberta and eastern Ontario expressed weight concerns. When they did, masculinity was reinstated through references to health, indirectly eschewing the feminine emphasis on weight loss for appearance or improved body image. One exception to this trend was André Aiken (fifty-five, white, upper middle class), an Athabasca County man who, after describing a childhood of "over-feeding" by his mother, used feminine language in referring to himself as "not very trim." In the main, however, more teenage boys than men expressed body image dissatisfaction in a classically feminized way, perhaps reflecting the fact that boys outnumbered men in the study.

As illustrated by Aarya Esani above, most boys shared adult male attitudes to dieting – weight loss and maintenance were not constantly on their minds, and they were generally blasé regarding body image issues. Embodied disciplinary techniques were not integral to their identities as they were for girls. For example, when asked whether or not weight was of concern to him and his friends, Alarik Eichmann (seventeen, white, lower middle class) stated, "Joking about it, but not really ... There's a lot [out there] about that, but I don't really care about it." When asked whether any of his friends experienced stress about their weight, he replied, "Not stressing. We joke about it, but we don't care."

Austin Enman (fourteen, white, working poor/impoverished) related a similar lack of concern about body weight among boys, characterizing the issue as a "girl thing": "Girls always think they're fat. At my school, they always think they're fat." When the interviewer asked, "Is body image then something that is talked about at your school?" Austin replied, "With the girls more. The boys don't really care that much. They're just, like, 'I don't care.'"

However, like some of the men, boys could be interested in "being healthy" through weight maintenance and weight loss, but their attitude differed from that of the girls and women. For example, Kris Keeshig (fifteen, First Nations, working poor/impoverished) had recently lost weight but did not characterize it as intentional or as vital to his identity: "I used to eat all the time; that's why I'm as big as I am, but I'm getting smaller and smaller." When asked what lay behind this change, he said, "Just not being hungry and more active and always out and about and no time to eat.'

Arlen Evans (eighteen, white, upper middle class) expressed an equally understated attitude toward weight:

> There's a difference between not wanting to be fat and actually caring what you – because it's pretty easy not to be fat. Just do some exercises. So, like, I don't actually work out, but I play soccer two times a week, and I try to eat healthy. Like, I'm not actually worrying about my figure, but I do my best to eat healthy.

Kolby Colwell (thirteen, white, working poor/impoverished) acknowledged the importance of weight maintenance through its potential impact on prowess in sports, a rather masculine framing. Thus, boys and men tended to relate to obesity and weight loss through the discourse of healthy eating, particularly through and for sport. This enabled them to perform weight-loss and maintenance regimes without appearing feminine.

A few boys, however, employed language and referred to experiences that are typically understood as feminine. For example, Arlen Evans articulated his weight maintenance regimes through exercise and sport but when asked whether he knew any boys who "care about their bodies," he stated, "I know a couple. I mean, every guy doesn't want to be fat." Kurt Comeau (sixteen, white, working class) suggested that boys did engage in weight-loss regimes but in a relatively covert way, especially in relation to their peers: "I think some guys will watch weight, personally, like they'll sort of think to themselves about doing it and try to do it at home, but when they're with their friends, it's sort of they just eat whatever. That's what I think ... [It's a] peer thing." When the interviewer suggested that "it wouldn't be so cool to say that" you're watching your weight, Kurt responded with a simple "No." Thus, he related important insights about the pressure on boys to manage their weight and to retain displays of masculinity through concealing practices regarded as feminine.

A few teenage boys dealt with feminized body image issues in everyday ways. Kim Kwan (eighteen, Chinese Canadian, upper middle class) was concerned about his recent weight gain at university:

> When I first entered university, they always told me about, like, the – what is it, the freshman fifteen or something? Lose fifteen minutes, gain fifteen pounds. And, like, actually the first few months, I didn't really gain any weight, so it's, like, "Okay, I'm fine." But now my pants are getting tight. Either [I need to] exercise more or eat better. Or the combination, I think.

Kolby Colwell (thirteen, white, working poor/impoverished) and his friend Keith, who joined his interview, were also interested in fitness and weight. In comparing their bodies to those of peers, and in taking up the language of eating disorders and "putting on pounds," they spoke in typically feminine ways:

> KOLBY: I'll admit that I eat a little bit too much junk food every
> once in a while, like, on the weekends mainly. And I'm

tall, but I'm kind of not as fit. Yeah. But we eat healthy, but we're not like – 'cause we've got some of our friends that are, like, anorexic. Like [our other friend], he doesn't gain a single pound.

KEITH: He can eat as much candy as he wants.

KOLBY: And he'd put on maybe a pound.

KEITH: Like, he'd have to eat it for a month, straight candy and nothing else, and then just gain one pound.

Self-surveillance and monitoring other people are apparent in Kolby and Keith's remarks.

Although parental pressure regarding weight generally targeted girls, boys were not necessarily exempt from it. This was evident in the Esani case study, where Adeela Esani criticized the "obesity" of her son Aarya. Mothers were more likely than fathers to worry about the weight of their sons. Like Adeela Esani, Amelia Albert (forty-one, white, lower middle class) related her anxiety about her son, Arthur (fourteen): "He's not eating as much as he had, which makes me happy. I'm getting concerned about his weight. He's fourteen, so how do you approach that? And he's really sensitive about his weight – I already know that. Six foot one already. And 253 pounds."

Some fathers were troubled about their sons' weight. As was the case for mothers and daughters, this was sometimes enmeshed in their own issues about identity and body image. For example, Andrew Albert (forty-one, white, lower middle class) expressed sentiments much like those of his wife, Amelia, in discussing their son, Arthur:

Well, as you've seen, my boy's a larger boy, and he does eat a lot as well, and I think his problem is the same as mine. That it's so good that I just want more, and then I'm still craving that, because it's been a while since we've had it, so I'm going to eat as much of it as I can right now.

One important gender difference was evident in the sample: unlike girls, boys did not articulate a clear opposition to body image issues as a macro-level discourse. They resisted pressures to diet and exercise on the individual level, as Aarya Esani repelled familial urging to lose weight, to eat "healthy" foods at home, and to exercise, despite prodding from his mother. Nor did boys express contempt for media representations of unrealistic body shapes and sizes. Although it is difficult to explain why, we do not attribute this lack to the absence of an idealized male body propagated in the media, as it certainly does exist (de Souza and Ciclitira 2005). It is possible, however, that the feminist counter-discourse to feminine body ideals has become so widespread and common sense that the female participants in our study could identify dominant beauty ideals with some ease. As yet, no such counter-discourse has been popularized for men or boys, perhaps because conversations about their weight are wrapped tightly (hidden, even) in discourses regarding health, strength, and sport, in order to be tolerable. Despite the experiences of boys in our study, dieting and weight maintenance to achieve a particular look remain largely outside mainstream assumptions regarding the behaviour of a "real" man.

CONCLUSION

Clearly, body image and weight issues remain central to the everyday lives of women and girls, many of whom critique weight maintenance even as they adopt it. This pattern is facilitated in part by the rearticulation of dieting as "healthy eating" within the wider fears of obesity as a rampant problem. Obesity narratives may even exacerbate disordered eating among women and girls (see Beausoleil 2009), in that they justify a set of behaviours that might normally be deemed unhealthy and sexist. The obesity panic also seems to be affecting male attitudes to body size, as was demonstrated by male interviewees who were concerned with weight and healthy eating, and especially by the teenage boys who approached body image issues in heretofore feminine ways. Though social pressures remain targeted particularly at women and girls, boys, too, engaged in self-governance and moral regulation through bodily surveillance and monitoring.

Our study does suggest that gender expectations concerning the body may be changing somewhat due to prevalent beliefs about obesity. Given (debatable) understandings of obesity as a state of ill health that decreases life expectancy (for an alternative perspective, see Flegal et al. 2007; Biltekoff 2013), gendered practices of fat avoidance are shifting, as dieting for both health and appearance seems to be increasingly available to teenage boys, even if it is undertaken discreetly. As this chapter shows, maintaining attractiveness has been deemed "women's work," but maintaining a "healthy weight" is increasingly everybody's job, regardless of gender.

6

social
class trajectories

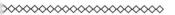

Noreen Hardie

NOREEN HARDIE IS a white thirty-eight-year-old who lives with her children, Neal (thirteen) and Nicia (nine), and her partner, Norbert Harrison (forty-four), in an affluent part of Halifax. Norbert's daughters from a previous marriage, aged nine and twelve, spend alternate weekends at the house, and Neal and Nicia spend every other weekend with their birth father.

Noreen has experienced a significant upward trajectory in her social class. She grew up on a farm in rural Nova Scotia, in a family she describes as "poor." Whereas her parents had less than high-school education, she earned a graduate degree and works full-time in health promotion. After a first marriage and divorce, she was a single parent for a time. Two years before our interviews, she moved in with Norbert, a surgeon, whereupon her household income increased to approximately $420,000 annually (about four times the Halifax median). We categorized her family as upper middle class.

Noreen is passionately committed to healthy eating and healthy living. Her family of origin grew, hunted, and gathered all its food, which she considers particularly healthy: the food is fresh, homemade, local, and organic. For Noreen, healthy eating is a moral virtue, a self-evidently better way, and she disparages unhealthy foods. She is proud that her children "have never known white bread and white pasta and all those types of things." Though she scorns certain foods for health reasons, many are associated with lower-class status and limited financial means. For example, she was horrified by the lunches that children brought to school in the lower-income neighbourhood where she lived as a single mother:

> Kids would bring, like, a little mini pop. I mean, it was just horrible ... little bottles, little Chubby's they're called, pop, like cream soda. There's just not, I mean no balance ... I volunteered to go on a field trip with them, and every kid had to bring a snack and a drink ... Cinnamon rolls and those Vachon cakes. I haven't even seen them for years! One guy had an extra-big Coffee Crisp and a pop. And his dad was there on the field trip, and I remember thinking "Oh my God, this is just awful!" I couldn't believe it.

In the neighbourhood where she currently lives, children bring very different lunches to school: "Kids had, like, sushi and cut up – you know a thing of grapes and a thing of snow peas and whole wheat pita and hummus. It's really so different." She obviously sees these lunches as nutritionally superior and more aligned with her own ideas of healthy eating. She is also delighted that she doesn't have to educate her daughter's new friends about healthy eating, because they "are not asking for white bread. They are not sticking their noses up about vegetables."

Noreen's approach is a good fit with her new upper-middle-class neighbours. However, she also holds tightly to the virtue of frugality when purchasing food. She attributes this to her childhood poverty, reinforced by years of financial constraint as a single parent. Noreen's healthy eating and frugality sometimes conflict with each other; for example, though she believes that organic produce is healthier, she decries the high price. Moreover, her thriftiness does not fit well with her new partner or lifestyle:

> I'm really frugal when it comes to eating as well. And that drives Norbert crazy. I think because I grew up so poor and then not having a lot of money as a single parent, I still really – I try to buy in bulk, I mean I never buy single-serving chicken; I always buy the biggest package you can. I'm constantly comparing prices, like how much it's going to cost per kilogram or per unit. He wouldn't do that in a million years. It's just very different backgrounds, right? He would just buy what he wants.

Cost is a main determinant of Noreen's decisions about food. At one point, she said, "I'm in budget mode. And that's probably, that's how I was raised. And that's how I will always be." Later, she added, "I will always be frugal. You'd swear I grew up in the Depression!" Such comments show how deeply her thriftiness is ingrained. Noreen remarks that she doesn't "believe in wasting money on anything" and gives no indication that she wishes to change this aspect of herself, despite the difficulty of balancing it with health, quality, convenience, and ethical eating, and the conflict it creates with Norbert, whom she sees as spending irresponsibly.

The upward shift in her family income means that Noreen has access to more expensive, higher-quality foods and specialty shops. Yet, she seems to need to justify her new shopping practices, emphasizing cost-effectiveness, quality, and avoidance of waste:

> They're pricey, yeah, but I just find some of their produce is so much nicer ... You go to the Superstore and there's nothing worse than spending all that money on Granny Smith apples, and then they're just mushy ... When I was a single parent, I definitely wouldn't have gone to a place like Pete's Frootique. To me that's a bit of a treat, because the prices are higher. The quality's really good.

Noreen and her family eat out at least once a week. Her two favourite restaurants are both fairly expensive, and she seems to justify the cost by emphasizing their ethical commitments, with local, organic, whole foods. Whereas she describes Norbert as caring most about the atmosphere of a restaurant, her focus is on food origins, quality, taste, healthfulness, and mode of production, which override her usual frugality. She downplays expense, emphasizing quality and ethics: "You feel like, wow! You are supporting an organization that is so progressive and buy only locally and all organic."

· · · *Netty Howell*

NETTY HOWELL, A white sixty-two-year-old, lives with her youngest son, Nolan (eighteen), in a subsidized housing cooperative in Halifax. Three years before our interviews, and after more than two decades of working as an alternative health care provider, Netty resigned due to health reasons and now relies on social assistance. Nolan, who had recently graduated from high school, is working at a grocery store before starting college.

Netty was raised in a middle-class family. Her parents had university degrees, her father worked full-time, they owned a car and a home, and they took summer holidays. Netty has completed some post-secondary education. Her ex-husband has a university degree, as do her two older children, and she describes her friends as professionals with master's degrees. Yet her social assistance income is approximately $8,000 per year, and we categorized her family as working poor/impoverished. Her class status has dropped significantly.

Netty is utterly committed to eating high-quality, locally grown, organic, mostly vegetarian food and strongly opposes the conventional agri-food system, which she views as unwholesome, environmentally destructive, and unsustainable. She developed strong views about the food system in the 1960s, when she adopted a back-to-the-land lifestyle. She sees her food decisions and practices as ethical acts that are fundamental components of her identity: "For me food is part of what I call wholesome sensuality. You know, a beautiful part of being is food and preparing it and eating it and feeling good from it and know how connected it is to sustaining our well-being."

Netty's interviews were filled with frustration about her current income level and the great difficulty of affording foods that were central to her sense of identity. Food is constantly on her mind, especially at the end of the month when money is tight. She spoke about going to bed worried about food. She is frequently unable to buy what she needs and rarely able to buy what she wants: "Do I need to borrow money for this? There's constant borrowing and then paying back."

When her money runs out at the end of the month, Netty uses a credit card to buy groceries, or she and Nolan confine themselves to beans and rice. There is considerable stress in the household, and the Howells' social lives are constrained by poverty. Netty rarely invites anyone to her home and feels guilty that she no longer allows Nolan to bring his friends over, because they empty her cupboards in minutes. When Nolan eats at the homes of "rich kids," she feels ashamed and fears that the parents will think "Oh, here comes that poor kid who has no food at home, cleaning out our cupboards." She worries about Nolan being hungry, expressing guilt about whether he is "getting enough": "Certainly not as much as he needed and not as much as ideally I would have fed him ... He should have had meat on the table every night and he didn't ... Lots of teenage boys wouldn't want beans and rice every night."

Despite her poverty, Netty almost always buys more expensive ethically produced food: "If I were baking and in a hurry, I might go to the Superstore, but I wouldn't buy anything but an organic flour." She prefers to buy from the producers themselves or small vendors rather than chain stores, even if it costs more and is less convenient: "I'd rather support small businesses. I believe that. I still believe – I know it's counter to the economic mentality, but there's more to life than economics."

Netty has occasionally used the food bank, but she scorns the quality of food provided as an insult to her dignity and now refuses to go there: "I am not interested in stale white bread; I won't eat it. I won't eat it! I'm not interested in packaged foods. I'm interested in fresh vegetables ... A typical day when I've gone in there, I've come home with all non-perishable foods ... It's not going to fill my relationship with food." In this relationship, food is a sensual pleasure, something to enjoy, to learn about and talk about. Netty described making pumpkin pies from scratch, using fresh pumpkin rather than canned, because, "There's a difference in how I feel making it. I take joy in making it. And it's just a whole process, that's the whole thing. Eating isn't just swallowing food."

Netty undertakes childcare to earn extra money for food. She occasionally uses food to demonstrate that poverty does not define her. For instance, she made an elaborate meal for visiting relatives, well beyond her financial means:

It still satisfied me to prepare and eat it. A lot of vegetables ... I brought the meat in as an expensive luxury for the company. And even the dessert was sort of luxurious for the company. And it wasn't to impress my brother as much – because my family knows who I am – as much as to honour them. You know, with sort of extra – at parties I spend more.

Experiencing income assistance as "humiliating," Netty distances herself from the food practices of other low-income families, whose diets she considers "despicable" because they include highly processed foods: "I know people on low income who buy a lot of bologna and hot dogs and I don't even know what they're called, but canned meats and things." She even castigates a well-off local family for unhealthy eating: "When I saw what they ate over at their house, I wasn't impressed, okay. Certainly, they were spending a lot of money on food. Lots and lots of money. Lots of boxed food, prepared foods, snack foods."

In contrast, Netty aligns herself with counterculture ways of eating. She has extensive knowledge of food production, distribution, and marketing, as well as nutrition and ethics. She knows all the nearby vendors of organic, local, and sustainable products, including the owners of food delivery programs and a small food co-op. Although she patronizes farmers' markets, she sees them as pretentious, "full of the upwardly mobile people" who have bought into a commercialized way of living that she scorns. For Netty, adherence to the dominant ethical eating approach, described in Chapter 2, seems paramount to confirming or conveying her former class identity.

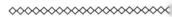

SURVEY RESEARCH FROM Western industrialized nations consistently shows that members of higher social classes conform more closely to dietary guidelines (they eat more fresh fruit and vegetables, lower-fat dairy products, and less fat overall, especially animal fat). Interestingly, however, nutrient intake does not significantly differ between classes (Power 2005). Clearly, class affects how people eat – most obviously in material ways, through how much they can spend on food, but also symbolically. In this chapter, we seek to understand how class affected participants' food practices and how they used food to mark symbolic boundaries, especially moral boundaries that display virtue and cultural and economic capital or class.

THEORETICAL FRAMING
Sociologist Pierre Bourdieu (1984) is particularly helpful in thinking about class and food practices. He identified four main forms of capital: economic (money and wealth), cultural (formal and informal education), social (relationships), and symbolic (honour, prestige, or recognition). Bourdieu understood social classes as reflections of the total "volumes" of capital held by individuals or groups, as well as the composition of the capital, especially economic and cultural. One kind of capital can be converted to another in processes of social class trajectory. So, for example, Noreen Hardie's cultural capital (her graduate education) and partnership with Norbert (social capital) brought economic capital, an upward class trajectory, and the symbolic capital

of living in an affluent neighbourhood. For Netty Howell, divorce (loss of social capital) brought a decrease in economic capital and the negative symbolic capital and shame of living on income assistance.

Symbolic capital carries value only when it is legitimated by the dominant class. So, for instance, healthy eating (see Chapter 1) holds symbolic capital because it is prized by the middle class. However, eating an unhealthy diet is not simply lacking in symbolic value; it is roundly condemned by the middle class, which sees it as disgusting. Thus, it carries a negative symbolism or stigma. In the case study above, Netty can be seen as distancing herself from the stigmatized identity of being on income assistance by drawing on the symbolic capital of the ethical eating repertoire (see Chapter 2), which is valued by members of the middle class, those whom Netty saw as her true peers.

As mentioned in the Introduction, we employed Bourdieu's concept of the habitus, in which social structures such as gender and class "get under our skin" to affect both our understanding of the world and our behaviour. The primary habitus of childhood is the most durable, probably because it is the least conscious. A tension can arise when habitus differs from current class location, a dynamic that Bourdieu (1984, 142) called *hysteresis*. The two case studies above are illustrative of this process, though both are extreme, possibly because Noreen and Netty experienced their economic changes relatively recently. For participants who had more time to adjust, the effects of hysteresis may have been more subtle. As we will see, some interviewees who experienced upward mobility appeared to have jettisoned their class origins in embracing the food practices of their new social location, whereas others brought their primary habitus with them, again without apparent hysteresis.

According to Bourdieu, all social practice has a logic, no matter how "illogical" it may seem to outsiders. The "logic of practice" relates to an individual's class position and to the amounts of capitals available to him or her. For those whose economic capital is small, finances often drive everyday decisions, leaving little room to exercise choice. Within this "logic of necessity," shopping for food generally focuses on avoiding hunger and getting the best value for the money spent. However, though poverty and economic hardship profoundly shape food culture, working-class tastes are not defined *solely* by restraint, restriction, and lack (see Bennett 2011), as will be clear in our discussion of frugality.

Those who enjoy a greater economic distance from necessity, with greater economic and other forms of capital, are more likely to develop a food culture that has an "aesthetic disposition," one in which food is seen not as "fuel," but as an arena of stylistic distinction, interpretation, and appreciation (Bourdieu 1984). Privileged populations tend to feel comfortable in a consumer culture and feel entitled to all that it has to offer, including its many food choices. At the same time, an upper-middle-class habitus entails the propensity for continual striving and disciplined self-improvement, such as an ongoing pursuit of health. Within this logic of "distance from necessity," the choices and practices of those who are closer to necessity may be rejected as unappealing.

Upper-class choices and practices are generally legitimated by the dominant culture and assumed to reflect superior taste and virtue. Thus, everyday behaviour can signal symbolic capital and mark boundaries between classes (Lamont 1992; Lamont and Molnár 2002). Such boundaries tell us, and others, who we are and who we are not. They differentiate classes in terms of hierarchy, inclusion, and exclusion. Thus, they can consign members of lower classes to less of everything that is valued by higher classes, including less taste, less intelligence, less virtue, less respectability, and ultimately less humanity (Lawler 1999, 2005). Hence, food practices can operate to maintain and reproduce social inequalities, even when the food culture is seemingly democratic and open to all (Johnston and Baumann 2010). It is important to note that symbolic and moral boundary marking is multidirectional; the lower classes, too, distinguish themselves through particular moral virtues. In the case studies above, both Noreen and Netty displayed alignment with middle-class virtues invested in healthy and ethical eating. Noreen, however, also prided herself on frugality, a quality she claimed from her working-class roots.

PARTICIPANTS, PLACES, AND APPROACH TO ANALYSIS
As was outlined in the Introduction, each participating family was categorized in terms of social class (upper, upper middle, lower middle, working, or working poor/impoverished) based on income, education, and type of employment. In sixteen households, one or more adults

had experienced significant downward or upward class mobility. Focusing on these families and the tensions that hysteresis can cause helps us make sense of food practices.

The sixteen families were from Vancouver, Edmonton, Kingston, Prince Edward County, Halifax, South Parkdale, and North Riverdale. Six had upward trajectories to the upper middle class. Seven had downward trajectories: five had become working poor/impoverished, one was now working class, and one was lower middle class. Three families had mixed trajectories: one moved from lower middle class to working poor/impoverished and then to working class; one transferred from lower middle class to working poor/impoverished and back to lower middle class; and one moved from working class to upper middle class, remaining in this class in occupational status but with a significant loss of income after divorce. Participant status changes are identified as follows: "U" indicates an upward trajectory, "M" a mixed trajectory, and "D" a downward trajectory.

In a pattern that is typical for Canada, all the upward trajectories involved some combination of education, employment, and marriage. As illustrated by the case study, Noreen Hardie's education, significantly beyond that of her parents, led to employment with a greater income. She later moved into a still higher class through her partnership with Norbert Harrison. The downward trajectories were also typical patterns, as illustrated by Netty Howell, who had less education than her parents, was a divorced single mother, and who had experienced unemployment due to a chronic health condition. The families with mixed trajectories conformed to this pattern as well; all three were headed by single mothers whose altered circumstances were related to divorce and changes in employment. In this chapter, we excluded families whose trajectory seemed mostly due to immigration, such as those who were upper middle class in their country of origin but underemployed in Canada. In these cases, the multiple reasons for changes in food practices, and ways of talking about food, were too complex to be analyzed solely in terms of class. They are featured in Chapter 8.

CLOSENESS TO NECESSITY: PRAGMATISM AND FOOD

Some participants saw food as a utilitarian necessity. This included almost everyone who had experienced downward mobility and were currently low income, and others who had moved upward but who retained a frugal habitus. For example, Tihana Raskovic (forty-eight, Serbian Canadian, upper middle class, U) attributed her pragmatic approach to food to her upbringing by immigrant parents who had little money: "Food is, to me it is a necessity ... I never would in my mind waste money frivolously on things that we really didn't need, but focus on what we did need. Like, always get your milk, your bread, your meat, your vegetable, et cetera. The fancy cakes, well, we'll save that for your birthday, kind of thing." Participants who shared this approach tended to apply it to the various tasks of feeding the family, including shopping and cooking.

Shopping as Task: Efficiency and Budget

For participants with an upward trajectory who exhibited a pragmatic habitus, shopping was a task to be accomplished as efficiently as possible. Despite their economic resources, these individuals valued convenience and tended to avoid patronizing multiple stores or specialty shops. For example, Avery Evans (fifty, white, upper middle class, U) was very clear that shopping was not a pleasure: "It's just, like, 'Oh God, I have to go grocery shopping,' and I just hate it. So it's just, like, you go to Safeway because you know where everything is ... I don't go to four other places ... I'm just not that kind of a shopper." Similarly, Tihana Raskovic avoided the farmers' market, which carried a wide range of specialty products, saying, "I just want to go and get food." These participants chose convenient grocery stores that sold a variety of items. When they shopped in several stores, it was to take advantage of sales and find the best prices, or what Tanya Pearce (forty-nine, Dutch Canadian, lower middle class, D) described as "chasing sales."

For six families with downward class trajectories and two with mixed trajectories, food shopping was based not on whim, want, or desire, but rather on need, budget, and cost. As Belinda Veitch (forty-nine, Scottish and First Nations, working poor/impoverished, D) said, "To be really honest, nearly all of our decisions are financially motivated. I'm on social assistance disability, so our food choices are according to what our finances are at that time." April Enman (forty-four, white, working poor/impoverished, D) planned family meals around what was on sale: "I'll go buy whatever's on sale; then we work around that, right?" What chanced to be on sale would even "dictate what we'll have for a treat." Others mentioned simply being unable to afford treats.

Following a budget was central to the pragmatic approach. Katrina Kellough (forty-six, white, working poor/impoverished, D) said, "You have to do the monthly budget – this is for bills, this is for gas, and here's what you have left over, and it has to do." Bronwyn Vale (forty-one, white, lower middle class, M) had begun using a budget for food shopping shortly after separating from her children's father: "What I found is just by meal planning, I could shave almost a couple of hundred dollars off my budget every month." She still shopped with a list and a calculator. Similarly, Kristi Keller (thirty-nine, white, working poor/impoverished, D) did mental addition as she shopped, so as not to exceed her food budget: "I add as I go ... If I get to fifty dollars and there's something that I need, like, I'll have to prioritize it. Then I'd take something out and put something back. And I can come within a dollar, a dollar fifty." These participants had extensive knowledge of food prices, and two mothers emphasized that they were teaching their teenaged children to comparison shop by price.

Some participants met their budgets by using a list. Anything not listed was not purchased. Bronwyn Vale made a weekly list before she went shopping:

> I sit down on the Sunday and I make a list of all of the dinners that I want to cook. So I usually use my cookbooks to do that. And then I take a look through my cupboards and see what I've got in the way of ingredients, and what I don't have I make up a grocery list. So I'm a list shopper.

If an item did not appear on her list, Bronwyn did not even enter its section of the grocery store. Netty Howell, from the opening case study, had multiple lists: what was desperate, what was needed, what she could actually afford to buy.

Some participants, including three with upward trajectories, used sales flyers and coupons to reduce cost. For instance, Katrina Kellough knew exactly when the flyers came out and embarrassed her children by shopping with coupons. She also took flyers to stores that would match the prices of other stores, a measure that saved her the time and work of "chasing sales" from store to store. Other participants, including Noreen Hardie in the case study above, bought sale items in bulk and froze the extras.

Some interviewees knew when each store put its products on the discount shelf, which enabled them to take advantage of the cheaper prices. For example, Keira Karsten (thirty-two, white, working class, M) always bought reduced-price meat and bread:

> We know when the meat is reduced, like, if you get there at 9:30, 10:00 in the morning, they have their meat reduced. We never pay full price for meat ... Mondays are the best day of the week to get the reduced meat, because they've reduced from the week-end what hasn't sold ... We never pay full price for breads or bagels, 'cause they've always got something there.

Participants who were close to necessity engaged in considerable work, much of it invisible, to ensure that they ate as best they could for the money they had. Although some took pride in their frugality, their shopping habits were shaped primarily by lack of money and were sometimes a source of shame and embarrassment for children.

Cooking as Necessity

For those with little distance from necessity, cooking was rarely used to display capital or impress others, and therefore they had no need to be food connoisseurs. April Enman (forty-four, white, working poor/ impoverished, D) had learned to cook at home, which she thought limited her range:

> My mom grew up on a farm, so pretty meat-and-potatoes and a vegetable ... So I probably watched her a lot doing that. We helped cook but she did most of the cooking. We probably learned more from just watching her. And didn't learn any ethnic cooking, though, at all. Like, it was all, like, roast beef or ham-burger, stuff like that. But nothing like ethnic cooking.

When these participants mentioned cookbooks, they were family cook-books. For example, Kristi Keller (thirty-nine, white, working poor/ impoverished, D) had her grandmother's cookbook: "I have her old recipe book, which is all in her handwriting. I have one from 1917."

For interviewees on low incomes, experimenting with new foods or preparation methods was risky. When asked how her eating might differ if she had more money, April Enman said, "I would definitely try out some different recipes ... A lot of times to buy all those ingredients, it's expensive and you're only going to use it once. So yeah, I would experiment a lot more with my cooking." Similarly, Ardith Elliott (fifty-five, white, working class, D) hesitated to experiment: "I'm not very adventuresome. If I'm going to cook, I'm measuring everything carefully, whereas I have a friend who just, 'Oh, you put some of this and put some of that.' I couldn't possibly cook like that because, partly because of the expense, because I wouldn't want to waste the money." Such pragmatism and cautiousness suggests little distance from necessity and little ability to use food for displays of capital.

Individuals who applied the pragmatic approach spoke about homemade foods not as artisanal treats prized for their authenticity, but more as taken for granted, normal, and consistent with their frugal orientation. For example, Tihana Raskovic had coveted friends' TV dinners as a child but later discovered that her homemade meals were much better:

> I grew up in an ethnic background, and I guess [with] our financial situation [you] did more, made more yourself. So in a way I used to feel deprived because other friends at school had Swanson dinners ... When I grew up, I tried the Swanson dinners and went ewwwww. But to me that was exotic, right? 'Cause we didn't have them. Now when I'm older as I've come to realize what I grew up on was really good food.

Tihana and her family typically had dinner at home, rarely ate out, and took leftovers for lunches. She did not romanticize homemade foods or see them as a particular accomplishment: she simply described them as normal.

DISTANCE FROM NECESSITY: PLEASURE AND DISTINCTION

Some participants who were currently or previously in the upper classes developed what Bourdieu (1984, 50) termed an "aesthetic disposition" toward food, seeing it as a source of pleasure, adventure, connection, and discovery. They tended to employ the dominant mode of ethical eating and the connoisseur approach to cosmopolitan eating, which were detailed in Chapters 2 and 3. This was illustrated by Netty Howell, who, despite having little money for food, insisted that "eating isn't just swallowing food." Interviewees with an upward trajectory, who had the financial resources to turn a biological necessity into an aesthetic choice and a vehicle for displays of capital, typically saw food as pleasure. For instance, Brent Vernon (fifty-three, white, upper middle class, U) spoke about cooking as "really fun ... a very wonderful relaxing thing to do that has great pay-offs at the end as well because it's good tasting." In describing cooking, he spoke about flavours and "sensual pleasure."

Food as pleasure was most clearly articulated by Bronwyn Vale (forty-one, white, lower middle class, M), who noted that she and her brother were becoming "foodies," transitioning from what she termed a "Hamburger Helper household" (Johnston and Baumann 2010). She spoke of food shopping and preparation as an event, discussing food as a favourite pastime: "I visit my brother in the summertime. He's a foodie and so we spend a lot of time talking about ingredients and going to markets, and lingering at the farmers' market for a Saturday morning, and spending a Saturday afternoon cooking and a Saturday evening eating."

In both preparation and consumption, she was interested in the "flavours and textures and visuals of food," and contrasted her approach to that of her parents: "I think it was a bit of a rebellious reaction to the very utilitarian nature of food in my parents' household." Bronwyn added that she wanted her children to learn that food was not just about hunger or health, but was also fun and "a way to express yourself."

Shopping as Fun

Some participants saw food shopping not as a chore, but as a leisure activity. Netty Howell loved going to the farmers' market:

> Going to the farmers' market is kind of going to a food circus and a people circus, and I love it for that reason ... The farmers' market is an education; it's exciting and it's a real incentive to

look at local produce too. And also to be aware of what all
there is really available right here in Nova Scotia.

Similarly, Bronwyn Vale enjoyed visiting numerous specialty food
shops, describing shopping as a fun activity, a "destination":

> I'll find myself at Donald's Market maybe a couple of times
> over the course of a week to buy fresh things. And then there are
> times when we feel like little splurges and that's when we go to
> places like the Grotta del Formaggio ... which has amazing
> cheeses, and we're a bit of a cheese household. We love our
> cheeses. So we'll try a new different kind of cheese. Or we'll go to
> Fratelli's bakery. It makes me hungry just to think about it. And
> get some special treat there. And go to the deli on the Drive and,
> you know. So sort of make our shopping a bit of a destination,
> a bit of an activity that we're doing. And that's fun to do ... It's
> a bit of exploration and taste testing. It's a foodie experience
> for sure.

These participants saw food shopping as pleasure partly because
they paid primary attention to wants and desires, rather than need
or cost. For instance, Karla Cleveland (forty-two, white, upper middle
class, M) made no attempt to find sales or bargains; her shopping
was based on desire: "Often the impetus to shop is that I have a craving for a certain something ... I get a craving and I go shopping."
Brent Vernon, whose family was featured in Chapter 3, was most explicit about his lack of concern for cost, in describing a recent shopping trip: "I didn't think about cost. I simply thought about what
I was going cook with what I bought ... I simply said, 'I think I'm
going to roast a chicken, and I'm going to do this with that, and I'm
going to get this, that, and the other thing,' and that was it."
   These individuals also tended to shop in multiple specialty stores,
foregoing the convenience of a supermarket for the pleasure of finding
the right ingredient. Bronwyn Vale happily looked "all over the city
for a deli that has brisket in a certain cut" because her son wanted to
try cooking it. Any of these participants might frequent a produce
store, one or more health food stores, a farmers' market, a cheese shop,
a fishmonger, a meat market, a coffee shop, a bakery, one or more

delis, and a chocolate shop. In addition, several families had organic produce delivered through various farm-to-table programs.

Some interviewees displayed high cultural capital by possessing esoteric or specialized knowledge about food stores, including quality, ownership, history, and suppliers. They detailed precisely which businesses carried which exotic or unusual ingredients. Brent Vernon's extensive discussion of the cheeses he had purchased demonstrated not only an encyclopedic knowledge of food (see Chapter 3) but also his eagerness to search out the perfect foods:

> The little Crottin de Chavignol is really delicious. It's lovely ... It's a goat cheese and it's a French cheese, and it just has a lovely sharpness to it and sweetness. Really beautiful. They are six dollars each, and they are about this big ... There's this beautiful texture to it. It's approaching dry when it's in a form that I like. The interior has this almost – what would it be like? It's not chalky, it's not as dry as chalky, but there's this certain dryness to it that is really appealing. This is when I like them, about this age. If you let them really age, the outside becomes very gnarly looking and the inside becomes more liquid ... But this is the form I like it, right about at that point.

Cooking as Leisure

To bolster their esoteric knowledge, some participants made a point of citing their sources of information regarding food and its preparation, including books and television shows. Food was a focus of adventure and discovery. For example, Belva Vernon (fifty, white New Zealand Canadian, upper middle class, U) had taken cooking courses, "like Dubrulle Culinary Institute when it was around, some serious amateur courses. Read a tremendous amount." Bronwyn Vale had also taken cooking lessons and learned from recipes and television: "I did take cooking lessons actually as a kid too. On Thursday nights, I'd go to the high school when I was about ten and do a little bit of cooking classes there. But really, the skills that I have now in cooking are completely self-taught pretty much, just from reading recipes, watching the food network."

Several people emphasized that they were very open to experimenting with cooking, confident that whatever they tried would be a success. Displaying cultural capital through cosmopolitanism and omnivorousness (see Chapter 3), Brent Vernon expressed utter confidence regarding baking, trying "new things with abandon," and preferring to cook "Northern Indian food, Pakistani food, Iranian food, Mogul food, Southern Indian food, and Thai food." Bronwyn Vale reproduced dishes that she had encountered elsewhere, "and most of the time it works out pretty good." She even trusted her cooking experiments when entertaining guests:

> Whenever I have company over, I tend to try a new recipe, which is kind of risky *[laughs]*. Because it could flop and it could be terrible, but I'm a pretty good cook so I can usually pull it off ... I consider myself a bit of a foodie, so I like to try new ingredients or new ways of cooking or just something really yummy, succulent and that I can share.

Possessing distinctive cooking equipment was another way of exhibiting cultural capital. In talking about her proficiency in the kitchen, Karla Cleveland stated, "I know how to cut things properly. I have a chef's knife, so I've got the tools I need, and I know how to use them." Brent Vernon had celebrated his fiftieth birthday by buying himself an expensive Italian coffee maker. He and his wife frequently referred to the bread oven he had built, "a back yard, fire-stoked brick oven," inspired by examples they had seen in Greece. Building an oven specifically to bake bread for family and guests bespeaks considerable distance from necessity.

For these participants, food was much more than a basic biological requirement. It was a vehicle for self-expression and displays of cultural and symbolic capital associated with upper-middle-class status.

BOUNDARY MARKING: DISTANCING AND AFFILIATING

As mentioned above, food and eating practices can be used to draw moral boundaries that establish class positioning. As such, they are both classed *and* classifying. In marking such boundaries, people distance themselves from those whose practices they reject. At the same time, they affiliate with the practices of the group to which they wish to signal belonging, using food symbolically to present themselves as virtuous, respectable, or worthy in comparison to others. In creating such boundaries, our participants adopted two main approaches: some used the practices and moral dispositions of their class of origin to distinguish themselves from their current situation, whereas others did the opposite, using the practices and moral dispositions of their current location to distinguish themselves from their class of origin.

A few families showed no evidence of boundary marking. They did not disparage the food practices of Others and did not seem to think that their own practices carried symbolic value demonstrating moral worth. Most, however, regardless of class trajectory, distanced themselves from lower-class or "low-brow" food, which included soft drinks, fast food, processed meats, powdered milk, and margarine. Just as Noreen proudly stated that her children had never eaten products made with white flour, some interviewees also rejected other "white" foods such as white bread, white rice, and pasta made with white flour. Netty and others scorned Kraft Dinner, Hamburger Helper, hot dogs, processed cheese slices, and bologna. Although these items were dismissed for health reasons, it is worth noting that many are relatively inexpensive. Their rejection suggests a moral condemnation that may extend beyond the food itself to include the people who regularly consume it.

In stark contrast, few participants (only one with an upward trajectory) said that the low-brow foods were acceptable and normal in their households. Avery Evans (fifty, white, upper middle class, U) appeared most comfortable with this, recalling that when her husband started his business, "it was pretty rough" and adding "we lived on hot dogs and Kraft Dinner." However, she made no effort to distance herself from this practice by relegating it to the past: "We still eat lots of hot dogs. You know, we're pretty basic hot dog, hamburger, chicken and steak." When asked about Kraft Dinner, she replied, "Oh, yeah. That's a staple in our house. Yeah, if we need a quick supper or whatever, yeah." Avery was not apologetic about choosing these foods and did not seem to perceive them as "bad" or "lesser," but she was an exception in our sample.

Othering and the Healthy Eating Discourse

Although people did employ ethical and cosmopolitan eating to convey both their social status and their distance from lower-class foodways, this was most often accomplished through the discourse of healthy eating. Interviewees with all kinds of class trajectories employed the discourse in a number of ways to Other.*

Most participants with upward class trajectories proudly insisted that neither they nor their children ever ate fast food, declaring it "just awful." Some with mixed or downward trajectories did eat fast food, at least occasionally, but asserted that it was "bad" in some way, usually in relation to health: "Lately, lunch has been a McDonald's chicken sandwich ... which is really bad and I never feel good after I eat it" (Karla Cleveland, forty-two, white, upper middle class, M). Kristi Keller (thirty-nine, white, working poor/impoverished, D) mentioned that she sporadically ate fast food but spoke at length about her daughter's rejection of it: "I still will, occasionally, have fast food, whereas she will not touch it ... She has such an aversion to it."

Bronwyn Vale, whose trajectory was mixed, went out of her way to detach herself from the foods of her youth, which she saw as unhealthy and inferior to her usual diet. These included grilled cheese sanwiches, hot dogs, and burgers. After visiting her parents over Christmas, and eating foods she did not normally consume, she undertook a cleansing fast to detoxify her body, drinking only juices for three days. Asked what foods required such a cleanse, she cited low-brow examples:

> It's a lot of meat, you know, hamburger, meatloaf, white bread, which I don't eat even when I'm there ... I didn't want to imbibe the kinds of stuff that they had in their fridge. It's really dairy- and meat-based. Carbs, dairy, and meat. There's not a lot of fresh vegetables and what there is my dad tends to overcook and over-pepper.

Physically cleansing to detoxify after eating the foods of childhood seems an extreme version of using the healthy eating discourse to achieve distance from class of origin. At a symbolic level, it could be

· · · · · · · · · · · · · · · · ·

* A term popularized by Edward Said (1978), "Othering" refers to social processes or discourses through which groups exclude and subordinate those whom they perceive as unlike themselves. At its worst, Othering casts the excluded group as less than human and therefore deserving of scorn, exploitation, or even death, in the context of war.

seen as a purification ritual to remove the lingering stain of association with a lower class (Douglas 1966).

Some participants explicitly used talk of nutrition and healthy
eating to demonstrate moral superiority over the eating practices of
other classes. As mentioned above, Noreen Hardie (thirty-eight, white,
upper middle class, U) spoke with horror about children's lunches
in the low-income community where she lived as a single mother.
She seemed to use the healthy eating discourse to distance herself
from her previous class status. Though low income, Katrina Kellough
(forty-six, white, working poor/impoverished, D) had been a community outreach worker who educated others about healthy eating.
She seemed to go out of her way to demonstrate to the interviewer
that she was not like "those people" – others whose incomes were
low. She knew that food practices could be used to make judgments
but did so nonetheless:

> I worked with a lot of these people, and it's nothing negative
> against them – a lot of them, when I met them in the grocery
> store and I'd see, I'm like "Oh, my God!" I try to not purchase
> a lot of what I see that they would have, so in some aspects, yes,
> I would choose some better stuff than them.

She believed that parents in her neighbourhood fed their children "a
lot of the bad school snack stuff" because "they're just ignorant of
the label-reading skills," skills that she herself had acquired.

Belinda Veitch and her fiancé, Bruce Vincent (forty-five, First
Nations, working class), used the healthy eating discourse to distinguish themselves from the other low-income members of their community and to connect with traditional First Nations ways of eating.
They acknowledged the challenge of eating healthfully on a low income yet maintained that it was possible. Like Netty Howell, Belinda
strongly distanced herself from the eating patterns of others who received income assistance:

> Go across the street and up one block to the First Nations lady
> who's lived over there who, you know, has three kids and is
> living on social assistance? Her diet will probably be McDonald's,

processed cheese sandwich on white bread, and Kraft Dinner, wieners, hot dogs, and bologna sandwiches ... Just about zero vegetables. Just about zero fruits. Tons of sugar, ice cream. Pop ... First Nations people in this area, their eating diets are horrible, really, really bad.

Belinda and other participants seemed to use healthy eating as a form of cultural capital to mark a class-based moral boundary between themselves and Others. Achieving distance from those in lower positions implicitly relies on negative stereotypes of the poor as ignorant, lazy, cheating the system, uninterested in health, immoral, and lacking judgment and taste. For participants such as Katrina, Belinda, and Netty, objective criteria would place them in the social position from which they sought to distinguish themselves. Thus, they had to work hard to assert a moral boundary between "us" and "them."

Boundary Marking Close to Necessity: The Virtue of Frugality

For those who live close to necessity, the ability to use food as a display of virtue, respectability, or symbolic capital is limited. Generally, only one strategy is available to them: frugality. Participants spoke of their thriftiness with considerable pride, suggesting moral boundaries between those who were frugal (good) and those who were not (bad). The latter were depicted – usually implicitly – as wasteful, extravagant, or frivolous. All who took pride in their frugality came from the lower classes and subsequently experienced upward or mixed trajectories. In demonstrating their moral worth and dignity, they "made a virtue of necessity" while also dismissing as profligate and immoral the practices of those who were further from necessity.

As we have seen, Noreen Hardie was most insistent and very proud about her frugality as a shopper, seemingly needing to convey that though she now had considerable financial resources, she had not always had them and did not need them. For her (and others), thriftiness was deeply embedded as a self-evident virtue and marker of moral worth, unconnected to her material circumstances. Avery Evans (fifty, white, upper middle class, U) described both of her parents being raised in poverty with a lot of mouths to feed: "There was times when they just had potatoes ... Like, there was potato soup." She added, "As we were growing up, that's why you always tried everything … You don't waste it." Participants spoke of being excited by discounted prices on food.

Another aspect of pride in frugality was knowing how to feed people for less. Keira Karsten (thirty-two, white, working class, M) said, "My mother could make a chicken last five meals, ending in the soup, of course … She knew a good bargain and she could make it stretch." Tanya Pearce (forty-nine, Dutch Canadian, lower middle class, D) described making a chicken last for several meals for herself and her daughter:

> I bought a whole chicken … We had it for dinner on the Friday, and then we had leftover chicken yesterday. There's still some more, hoping to make, like, chicken salad sandwiches or something like that tomorrow. And I've saved the carcass to try to make soup. So I'm hoping by doing it that way, that's quite a few meals out of that.

Similarly, when some participants mentioned eating out, they focused on cost and value more than on food quality or cuisine. April Enman (forty-four, white, working poor/impoverished, D) shared her technique for ensuring that she got the discount price on buffet lunches. Kristi Keller highlighted portion size when naming her favourite restaurant, and Keira Karsten detailed one place where the meals were big enough to share and another where "the prices are fairly good for the portion sizes." She had also taken a course in Chinese cooking so that "we can have a Chinese meal at home that still is a six-course meal for under twenty dollars."

Boundary Marking through Ethics and Authenticity

Participants who were distant from necessity had numerous ways of differentiating between themselves and Others and of showing their affiliation with highly prized social locations. These included various elements of ethical and cosmopolitan eating. To distinguish herself from a lower location, Netty Howell employed the dominant mode of ethical eating, emphasizing upper-class values and priorities rather than cost and necessity. All her decisions about food were made through an "eating green" lens, and she also pointedly displayed encyclopedic knowledge about the food system, including citing several books during interviews. Most participants with downward trajectories employed a similar strategy, marking affiliation with their middle-class origins via the dominant ethical eating mode. In contrast, many upwardly mobile interviewees seemed unable to overcome their frugality to buy organic, fair-trade, sustainable, ethically produced foods. Noreen Hardie said, "When you look at organics, it's so much more expensive." Trent Payne (fifty-three, white, upper middle class, U) went further: "I'm still somewhat skeptical that the claims for organic are really, truly organic."

Most participants with upward trajectories also emphasized their affiliation with the connoisseur mode of cosmopolitan eating, stressing their receptiveness to foods from any ethnic cuisine and deliberately inculcating similar openness in their children. They highlighted the exotic, referring to little-known "hole in the wall," "one of a kind" places. As Noreen Hardie pointed out, "I find the best foods are often dingy little places like little Thai places, where they could care less about how things look or the tables are set up."

The upwardly mobile interviewees particularly signalled their affiliation with class elites through a quest for authenticity, quality, and taste, which marks a "foodie" approach to eating (Johnston and Baumann 2010). Interestingly, some proponents evidently needed to ensure that they were not perceived as elite, pretentious, or snobbish (an avoidance that is also part of high-status foodie behaviour) (ibid.). They attempted to render invisible the economic and cultural resources that were required to achieve this form of symbolic capital, perhaps because they came from lower-class positions where snobbery was often ridiculed (Bourdieu 1984; Lawler 1999).

Trent Payne, who said he was escaping his "lunch-bucket town" upbringing, disparaged foods that he associated with poverty, laughing about "onions and turnip and cabbage." Yet in talking about his current eating habits, he joked, "No caviar!" a quip intended to express his non-elitist attitude. Belva and Brent Vernon were even more explicit in distancing themselves from pretentiousness. They belittled a local restaurant as having "obsequious service" and being "over the top." When examining a photo of a restaurant, they also rejected it as "too stuffy" and overly self-conscious, remarking, "You couldn't put your elbows on the table and talk" and "You're wondering whether or not you've got the right wine glass." They adamantly dismissed what they called "epicureanism," or superficial knowledge of foodie fads:

BRENT: I think what's happened here in Vancouver in the last fifteen years is there's a greater epicureanism developing where discussions are about the most fabulous baguette to get. You can't just have normal bread ... There's a definite thing happening ... specifically in upper-middle-class Vancouver ... that is about having the best of the best ... It's just another aspect of increased consumerism.

BELVA: It's like yoga's popular now ... and then it will become, something else will be popular ... Things come and they go, and I think that's happening now with epicureanism ... It's unfortunate because it's superficial. It's about kind of ... being seen to consume the best. It's not about any kind of direct meaningful knowledgeable relationship with the food that's ongoing, that's kind of like a lifetime relationship that's deep and grows.

The Vernons carefully distinguished their own food practices, which they saw as authentic (a defining trait of foodie culture), from those closest to them, the "epicureans" who indulged in what they judged to be superficial fads. A casual observer might find it difficult to see the difference.

Among those who saw food as pleasure, quality and authenticity were perhaps most prized in homemade foods. These were idealized as inherently better, a distinction that enabled participants to distance themselves from the prepared and packaged foods of the lower class. As Trent Payne (fifty-three, white, upper middle class, U) said, "We don't eat almost any packaged food at all, like prepackaged skillet this or canned that." He went on to say of most packaged and fast foods, "I think we make way better ones, and you can make way healthier ones, at home." Similarly, when shown a photo of macaroni and cheese, Brent Vernon disparaged it because it looked prepackaged and said he would eat it only "if that were a macaroni and cheese like we can make ourselves." Noreen Hardie, who grew up on a farm but who now had a full-time job and a hectic urban life, spoke about home cooking and preserving in ways that were particularly romanticizing:

I wish I had more time to do it. I mean, ideally I'd love to just be working part-time and be home part-time, so I could put more energy into things like that. I love, I loved as a kid, picking berries. I love actually gathering food and bringing it home. You know what I mean? And then making the meal. I love the whole process.

Bronwyn Vale had once made preserves to sell at a farmers' market for extra money, and though lack of time now limited her output, she still gave them as gifts to friends and family. She preferred home-made foods, especially for company, because of their superior quality: "I like it to be all homemade, so you know homemade desserts and homemade appetizers and just you know – I don't, it's pretty rare that I'll buy a boxed something. Something pre-prepared. Because I want to be in charge of the flavours and the ingredients."

CONCLUSION

A key point in this chapter is that the connection between class and eating practices encompasses more than income alone. Those in differing class positions, with different trajectories, habitus, and distance from necessity will consequently apply different logics to their food practices, all of which are based in the material and cultural aspects of their lives and the symbolic capitals that arise from those contexts. Examining those whose past and present class locations were in tension enabled us to better understand the logic of their everyday eating, as well as the ways that food can mark class-based moral boundaries. When economic circumstances change, the habitus and dispositions learned in childhood could be difficult to discard. In particular, distance from necessity or proximity to it may result in a focus on food as pleasure or food as necessity. Several upwardly mobile individuals had adopted a pragmatic approach to shopping and cooking, whereas others who were currently living in poverty retained a deep sense of food as sensual pleasure and a means of expressing desires, politics, and adventurousness.

Food was used to mark boundaries, asserting distance from or alignment with certain class locations, as was particularly evident in the case of Noreen Hardie and Netty Howell. As Bourdieu (1984, 479) explained, "Social identity lies in difference, and difference is asserted against what is closest, which represents the greatest threat." Thus, those who feel shame in occupying a stigmatized class position must work hard to establish their distinctiveness from others in the same position. Those who have left a stigmatized class but still feel shame may attempt to distance themselves from it. Conversely, members of the middle class may "push away" lower-class practices with a vehemence that can only be described as disgust. Doing so helps to constitute and solidify their own positions (Lawler 2005).

Interviewees who prioritized ethics, pleasure, and adventure were drawing a moral boundary by promoting the superiority of their way of eating, while also signalling high economic and cultural capital. Their approach separated them from "mass," standardized, low-brow culture and the speed of modern life, distinguishing them from the lower classes, which treat food as a necessity. In contrast, those who stretched a meal or shopped for bargains claimed the superiority of a frugal approach, implying (if not stating) that anyone who dispensed with it was wasteful and frivolous.

— 7 —

movements
within canada

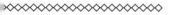

Trudy Patterson

TRUDY PATTERSON IS a white sixty-year-old who moved from Halifax to Toronto some forty years ago, though she still visits "home" often. She lives with her grandson Travis (seventeen), who is in high school, and she volunteers part-time and does community work. Her income is very low (below $20,000 annually, about half the local median), and thus we categorized her family as working poor/impoverished.

Trudy argues that food practices in Halifax are less healthy than in Toronto. For example, after migrating, she learned to drink lower-fat milk:

> Two percent milk now is okay. I find it's a little bit too creamy in my tea now, but I mean I'm fine with 2 percent and I'm fine with 1 percent. I actually enjoy a cold glass of 1 percent milk. So you change your eating habits, you know. You might be raised on homo[genized milk]. You know, in Halifax, Nova Scotia, we always had the can of Carnation Condensed Milk on the table to go in our tea. That's very thick and creamy, and to get down to 1 percent, you know, it's a healthier choice I would say.

Though some of Trudy's comparisons may concern changes over time more than distinctions between places, she argues that the two cities are also different currently: "When I go down to visit [Halifax], they all sort of eat the same." She finds that food is considerably more expensive in Halifax, which she cannot fathom, given the abundant farmland nearby: "My family's tired hearing me complain because every time I go, I'm criticizing in the grocery store."

She also praises the wider variety of foods in Toronto: "It's much more multicultural foods. Much more variety, much more accessibility of that variety. Prices are a lot better, so you can afford to buy a variety of foods." In multicultural Toronto, Trudy's food repertoire has broadened over time: "It wasn't even conscious, just gradually trying to expand a little bit and trying different foods ... I have expanded my repertoire to include foods that I wasn't raised up with, like pita bread." She eats spicy food such as tacos, as well as pasta and rice, which were not part of her upbringing: "My food choices have changed a lot, I guess being away from my family and not having that influence."

Nonetheless, there are limits to Trudy's adventurousness, which she attributes to her upbringing:

> I eat foods that I wouldn't eat as a kid ... In the culture that I was raised in, a meal would consist of meat and potatoes or fish and potatoes. We weren't pasta or rice people. With a vegetable. To me that's a meal; meat and potatoes and vegetables would be a meal ... That's sort of the way I was raised. My food choices have changed a lot ... but I'll still go out with people, and I won't try foods.

Trudy described a recent visit to a sushi restaurant with friends, where she found the food inedible: "It was just awful." She added that "there's still a lot of stuff I won't eat. Like mangoes." Though her approach to food is bolder than that of her family in Halifax, and certainly more so than in her youth, she still balks at completely unfamiliar dishes, displaying a tentative approach to cosmopolitan eating (see Chapter 3). She attributes her conservatism to her roots: "I guess there's still an influence from my culture growing up." Trudy does not seem particularly embarrassed or concerned about this, describing it matter of factly as part of her approach to food.

···*Karine Clements*

KARINE CLEMENTS IS a white fifty-one-year-old who was born outside of Montreal and was raised in Toronto from the age of seven. About eight years ago, after living in Toronto for approximately thirty years, she moved with her husband and two young children to Prince Edward County, Ontario. Karine is a music teacher, and her husband is a self-employed cabinet-maker. Their son just moved away from home, and their daughter, Kennedy (thirteen), is in Grade eight. We categorized the Clements family as lower middle class, with an annual income of about $33,000 – well below the community median but slightly above the cost of basic shelter, food, clothing, and transportation (see Table 1, page 20).

Like Trudy Patterson, Karine sees Toronto as a haven for cosmopolitan eating. She finds little opportunity for this in Prince Edward County: "We've always eaten a lot of ethnic food, which is also another thing, because a lot of things like Indian food and so forth, we really like. Mexican food, Indian food, Thai food. And that's something I have to say, out here, you can't get. I mean, unless you're going to make it yourself."

Karine takes a pragmatic approach to cosmopolitan eating (Chapter 3), enjoying encounters with a variety of ethnic cuisines, even seeking them out, though not emphasizing connoisseur knowledge and novel experiences. Ethical eating is the main food priority in the Clements household. The family is highly engaged with a dominant approach to food ethics (Chapter 2), focusing on local, sustainable, and organic products: "We eat a lot of organic food … We try to always buy fair-trade organic, always, as much as possible of everything we buy … We try and not eat too much packaged stuff." She and her husband have been vegetarian for twenty-five to thirty years. Karine loves Prince Edward County's easy access to fresh, high-quality, local, organic food:

> It's great here, as far as buying locally. We grow our own; we can get stuff from local vendors that we don't grow. You can get mushrooms at the mushroom farm. I mean, it's really amazing, anything, eggs, you don't have to go far. And last year … I was trying to eat on the hundred-mile diet for a month, and we wanted to get flour … and we found a place … an organic farm, and they grow wheat and various other specialty grains and oats and all that kind of stuff. And they have a mill.

Karine and her husband grow much of their own food, using organic techniques to enhance the soil. She emphasizes the politics embedded in food consumption choices, speaking at length about olive oil she buys from a Palestinian growers co-operative. During her interviews, she cited authors who had written books about ethical eating.

According to Karine, her family and friends eat differently from Prince Edward County locals: "In our circle, a lot of people eat like us ... They eat well ... They would be into having local, good food." In contrast, locals frequent McDonald's and are uninformed about "really good food." She attributes her distinct eating habits to her years in Toronto:

> In the city there's more diverse nationalities, first of all, so there's exposure. And there's more exposure to restaurants with really good food. And I'm not saying – I mean, we have a book club where we all love to bring food, and we have County people and newer people, and food's all great. And I like somebody's mashed potato casserole just as much as the next person *[laughs]*. But there are a lot of things – like, if you look at cookbooks from, say, the Women's Institute or a local church or whatever, you're gonna get some things that I personally wouldn't consider great food, you know? Jellied salads and, you know. I think that's a rural thing.

Focusing primarily on rural-urban difference, Karine describes local eating habits as relatively unsophisticated and concerned with quantity more than quality:

> You do get people who ... shop for quantity, and so they eat more of stuff, but it's not good stuff, you know? And possibly sometimes being more easily influenced by media maybe? You know, if they don't feel confident enough to cook themselves or ... if they just wanna buy a box of macaroni and cheese for sixty cents, it's just as cheap, and then they think, well why would I grow my own? It's a whole education thing.

Karine believes that home education is key to eating habits. She suggests that people in the County grew up watching their mothers make prepared food from boxes, which is what they know and like. As a long-term vegetarian, she thinks that local farmers might not understand the politics of raising animals for meat: "I'm not trying to offend them by not eating meat.

But I do think it's not a good thing. Feed lots and all that. But how do you tell someone who's done that all their – that's their whole life?"

An interesting tension appears in Karine's interviews; though she and her friends greatly value their access to the fresh, high-quality, local, ethically produced and distributed foods of the County, she does not believe that locals appreciate what they have or even what they themselves produce: "They make their own cheese and it's so good; they make artisanal-type foods and they don't even know that they are, if you know what I mean. They make awesome food and they don't even realize how special it really is. Like Pat's Jams ... She's always done it and it's awesome and it's really good."

As a vegetarian and ethical eater, Karine is thrilled with her new rural environment where fresh, locally grown organic food is widely available, but she does mourn the loss of easy access to diverse ethnic cuisines.

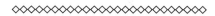

DRAWING ON INTERVIEWS with participants who had moved from one part of Canada to another, this chapter explores how they used discourses of healthy, ethical, and cosmopolitan eating to construct "places" and to constitute their own social identities in relation to them. People who have moved from one location to another may experience hysteresis, the disjuncture between the embodied preferences of their upbringing and those demanded in the new context (Bourdieu 1984, 142). Social and cultural patterns concerning food can become much more obvious when people travel or move to a new place, where suddenly they find themselves surrounded by people whose eating habits differ from their own. At the same time, food practices can be used to mark symbolic boundaries, distinguishing "us" from "them" (Lamont and Molnár 2002). Here we particularly focus on boundaries related to place – regional distinctions as well as urban-rural differences.

It is important to note that our focus is on how people talked about eating in a particular place, not on ascertaining the "truth" of the situation. Three people may live in Edmonton, but how they experience and understand its food may differ depending on whether they were raised there, migrated from a tiny village, or moved from a cosmopolitan city such as Toronto. We can explore how they use food practices in Edmonton to support or emphasize their own social identities and to construct an image of the city's foodways.

One challenge of this analysis is that when participants moved from one region to another, they often moved from a city to a more rural area, or from the country to an urban centre. Thus, what they saw as regional differences were often interwoven with rural-urban differences. Also, geographic mobility is often coupled with class mobility. When people speak disparagingly about food practices in the place they left behind, they may also be talking about a class identity they wish to jettison (see Chapter 6). In addition, migration sometimes occurred in the distant past, as we saw with Trudy Patterson. Participants might be comparing their current situation with that of years, or even decades, earlier.

THEORETICAL FRAMING

The geography and economic-political history of Canada feature regions at least as much as nation. Though its regions arguably exhibit as much diversity within as between, Canada is traditionally divided into six of them: the Atlantic Provinces (Nova Scotia, New Brunswick, Prince Edward Island, Newfoundland and Labrador); Quebec; Ontario; the Prairie West (Manitoba, Saskatchewan, and Alberta); British Columbia; and the North. Regional settlement patterns differed historically (McGillivray 2010), with European fishing vessels exploring the East Coast in the fifteen hundreds and permanent colonial settlements spreading from the east into Central Canada (Quebec and Ontario) during the sixteen hundreds. In contrast, the West Coast was occupied solely by indigenous peoples until well into the seventeen hundreds, and British Columbia became a British colony only in the 1850s. The Prairies were colonized by Europeans even later, after the completion of the Canadian Pacific Railway in the late 1880s. Whereas the British and French dominated the west and east, the Prairie settlers included many Eastern Europeans. The Canadian North still remains largely the domain of Aboriginal peoples.

Canadian regionalism also has economic and political roots. Central Canada has long been the economic "core" of the country, with the rest seen as the "periphery" (ibid.). During the eighteen hundreds, southern Quebec and Ontario became Canada's manufacturing heartland, enjoying easy railway access to both markets and raw materials from the "hinterland." An industrial economy developed in the centre, whereas that of the periphery was based on resource extraction – fish, furs, lumber, agriculture. The centre could think inclusively of a Canadian nation, but the periphery began to view it with suspicion, aware that, in selling resources cheap and buying products at considerable markup, it was essentially subsidizing Central Canada's economy (Harris 2012). Federal politics reinforced this core-hinterland divide, with governments elected by the populous Central Canadian provinces, whose interests often differed significantly from those of the periphery. Ongoing economic inequities among the regions helped to maintain regional identities (Corrigall-Brown and Wein 2009).

Regional Identities and Foodways

Identities are never static; they change with context. Nor are they singular; multiple aspects of an individual's identity constantly intersect. Particular identity markers recede to the background or rise to the foreground, depending on context. For example, identity for a Prince Edward Islander might centre on hometown or village; if that person moves to New Brunswick, being "an Islander" might be most salient; if he or she later moves to Ontario, being Atlantic Canadian might matter most. The salience of place-related identity changes with context.

Generally speaking, Canadians are more likely to identify in regional rather than national terms, particularly outside of Ontario (Hillier 1996; Corrigall-Brown and Wein 2009). Regional identities are not simply a product of economic-political history: they also arise from cultural differences and even stereotypes that become part of nationally articulated perceptions. Francophone Quebec is only the most obvious instance of this. British Columbia (at least its southern section) is often seen as populated by outdoor-loving, back-to-the-land hippy types, whereas Atlantic Canada may be seen as home to politically conservative, traditional, slightly backward but friendly people.

Although efforts to identify a Canadian national cuisine have proved largely unsuccessful (Pandi 2008; Kenneally 2009), elements of regional cuisines do exist (Hashimoto and Telfer 2006; Blue 2008; Tye 2008). Though none are unique to a single region, consider Atlantic seafood, Scottish-influenced oatcakes, Acadian rappie pie, fiddle-heads, molasses on biscuits, Newfoundland toutons, and PEI potatoes. Or Quebec maple syrup, tourtière, poutine, local cheeses, wild game, and cipaille. Or Ontario wines, apples, sausages, smoked meats, and "ethnic" foods. Or Prairie wheat, perogies, Alberta beef, bison, pemmican, and Saskatoon berries. Or BC wines, smoked salmon, Nanaimo bars, peaches and cherries, and Asian-influenced dishes. Or Northern Arctic char, seafood, caribou, muskox, seal, ptarmigan, and berries.

Food patterns and practices can be a significant part of creating and marking regional identities (Hashimoto and Telfer 2006). For example, Blue (2008) argues that Alberta beef symbolizes a regional identity in which Albertans are framed as political mavericks, distinct from the rest of Canada due to their social conservatism, Western alienation from Central Canada, and collective interest in oil and gas, as well as beef ranching. Alberta beef evokes images of cowboys riding the range on the Western frontier. Similarly, Tye (2008) suggests that molasses was once a staple in Atlantic Canadian households, especially those with little income. For those who have left Atlantic Canada, or who may remain there but are no longer living so close to the bone, molasses conjures "an imagined community with an imagined past when people worked hard and made do with what they had, even when that wasn't enough. Molasses carries proof of ingenuity and skill; people provided for themselves" (ibid., 345). Food can arouse nostalgia, a taste of home or of an earlier time at home. It can evoke an imagined home, even one that never existed or that no longer exists. Regional foodways are representations of a people, a place, and a time, and may thus be useful in marking boundaries of identity.

Urban and Rural Foodways

Most Canadians live in urban areas (81 percent), reversing the pattern of the past (Human Resources and Skills Development Canada 2013), and many recognize rural-urban differences in food practices. In public discussions, the portrayal of rurality is ambivalent (McPhail, Chapman, and Beagan 2013). Rural spaces are constructed as pastoral, idyllic places where people grow their own food with a kind of purity and traditional authenticity. This connects to a long-standing historical discourse about urban centres as defiling and degenerate (Thorpe 2012). At the same time, rural areas are frequently conflated with the working class and working poor, who are stereotypically imagined as uneducated and unsophisticated manual labourers. Rural-dwellers are portrayed as mired in tradition and unable to cope with the progress of modernity, leaving them backward and behind the times (Everett 2009). In contrast, urban environments are depicted as modern, progressive, and enlightened (Creed and Ching 1997); "the urban" is the assumed reference in most social theory, overlooking the logic of practice (Bourdieu 1984) of rural places.

Rural foodways are generally characterized as involving limited choice and access to fresh produce (Liese et al. 2007), with rural-dwellers relying on the modern food system like everyone else, rather than growing their own food. Isolation is understood as the main factor affecting their choices. Rural areas are also thought to have disproportionately higher obesity rates than urban centres (Mitura and Bollman 2004; Plotnikoff, Bercovitz, and Loucaides 2004; Bruner et al. 2008; Ismailov and Leatherdale 2010), due in part to lack of exercise, as farming has become more mechanized. In addition, stereotypes of working-class and rural people cast them as unaware of the supposed health benefits of avoiding obesity (Everett 2009). This perceived lack of sophistication is reinforced by a tendency to food conservatism in at least some rural districts. Rural-dwellers may attend more to tradition, balance, and the sociability of meals, leaving the desire for exotic and gourmet foods to urbanites (Lupton 2001).

PARTICIPANTS, PLACES, AND APPROACH TO ANALYSIS

The analysis for this chapter examined interviews with participants who had experienced significant moves within Canada – usually from one region to another, sometimes between provinces within a region, and a few (such as Karine Clements) between very different food environments in a province, such as from a major city to a rural area. The intent was to select interviewees who were most able to reflect upon the typical food patterns of an area, informed by having lived elsewhere.

In twenty-nine families, one or both adults had migrated within Canada. Three of the twenty-nine lived in Halifax, and at least one had grown up in Ontario or Quebec; five lived in Kings County, Nova Scotia, and at least one had grown up in Ontario, Newfoundland, or the North. Four families lived in Kingston, with parents who had lived throughout Canada; six families lived in Prince Edward County, with parents who had lived in Toronto, Montreal, Nova Scotia, and the BC West Coast. In Toronto, only two South Parkdale families fit the migration criteria, with adults who had lived in rural Ontario, Quebec, and Nova Scotia. One Edmonton family had migrated from Saskatchewan, and two Athabasca County families had moved from Victoria and Vancouver. In Vancouver, four families had relocated from Toronto, Alberta, and the North; two District of Kent families had moved from Vancouver Island and Saskatchewan.

Attempting to determine how participants talked about food in relation to place, our interviewers asked them, "How do people eat around here?" and "If someone was visiting and wanted to see how people from around here eat, where would you take them? What would you feed them?" We also asked, "How does how you eat now differ from the ways you ate growing up, if at all?" Throughout the analysis, we kept in mind that their responses could intertwine perceptions of region, class, rural-urban differences, and change over time.

DEPICTING URBAN FOODWAYS

Cosmopolitan Variety

Those who had moved to cities (particularly Kingston, Toronto, Edmonton, and Vancouver) generally gave glowing accounts of their cosmopolitan options, such as Trudy Patterson above. Kyra Kiernan (fifty-one, white, lower middle class), Kristi Keller (thirty-nine, white, working poor/impoverished), and Keira Karsten (thirty-two, white, working class) all depicted Kingston as a city that, for its size, had an unusual number of high-quality restaurants serving diverse cuisines. Kristi described its downtown restaurant scene as "local" and "alternative": "Restaurants, the wide variety, huge variety and excellent food. Just really, really good food. There's great Thai, Indian, there's Chez Piggy's, which is an entity unto itself." Virtually everyone who lived in Kingston mentioned Chez Piggy, which had influenced the local food culture for thirty years. As Kyra explained, before Chez Piggy came to town, the idea was that going out was prime rib, meat, potatoes, and if you're lucky you got fish ... And then Chez Piggy came along, and there are all these crazy Thai things mixed in with this, that, and the other thing. And people got a lot more adventurous. And now Kingston has an amazing variety of different places where you can go eat.

Adam Edward (thirty-seven, white, upper middle class) and his wife, Abby (thirty-six, white), had moved to Edmonton from small-town Saskatchewan ten years earlier and described it as far more cosmopolitan: "There's so many ethnic cultures here in Edmonton. There's German, Dutch, Indian, Chinese." Adam referred to a Polish bakery, a French restaurant, a very high-end steak house, and Edmonton's Chinatown. He thought there was also a "little Italy," though he was uncertain where.

In South Parkdale, Trent Payne (fifty-three, white, upper middle class) and his wife, Tina (fifty-one, French Canadian), had migrated from small-town Ontario and Quebec. Highlighting the availability of diverse foods, Trent said, "We just can get everything. We can get access to everything because of the multicultural neighbourhoods." They cited numerous examples of restaurants from every possible ethnicity, discussing the distinctions between Guyanese and Caribbean roti, between Thai and South Indian curry, and between Balinese and Polynesian food. They cooked meals from many of these cuisines.

Similarly, both Brenda Voisey (forty-nine, Irish Canadian, working poor/impoverished) and Bronwyn Vale (forty-one, white, lower middle class) emphasized the wide variety of foods available in Vancouver. Bronwyn saw the food of her Edmonton youth as far less cosmopolitan than that of Vancouver: "I never had ethnic food really much. Maybe the odd Chinese food dinner night with my parents, but when I was young it was pretty meat-and-potatoes. Sort of Alberta steak." Although Brenda's comparisons may also reflect the passage of time, she also made up-to-date comparisons. In contrasting the food preferences in her daughter's school with those of her nieces and nephews in Edmonton, she argued that even teens in Vancouver have cosmopolitan palates, comfortably eating sushi, roti, and samosas: "In Vancouver what teenagers eat is, I think, pretty broad compared to, say, if I went back to Edmonton, and my family has never had butter chicken. And yet, if you served it at my daughter Brogan's school, you'd sell out. I think it's regional." When the interviewer asked, "Teenagers have a more kind of international palate here?" she replied, "Yeah, absolutely."

Everyone agreed that Toronto and Vancouver were characterized by cosmopolitan food repertoires, but the view of Edmonton was less consistent. Bronwyn Vale and Brenda Voisey saw it as having narrow and conservative foodways, compared with those of Vancouver, whereas Adam Edward, who had migrated from small-town Saskatchewan, experienced it as highly cosmopolitan.

Halifax, Atlantic Canada's largest city, was consistently portrayed as lacking a cosmopolitan food repertoire. In her case study above, Trudy Patterson described her Halifax upbringing as having a narrow focus on the traditional meat-and-potatoes diet. Spicy foods, pasta, and rice, which were foreign when she was growing up, remained relatively off-limits among her family and friends in Halifax. Norma Horne (forty-five, white, lower middle class) had reversed Trudy's migration, moving from Toronto to Halifax. In Toronto, she ate out quite often, sampling a wide variety of ethnic cuisines, which she missed in Halifax. In discussing its "multicultural" cuisine, she said there was "a lot of Middle Eastern food" but added that it was mostly fast food: "Donairs are actually Lebanese in origin, and that's the provincial food isn't it? I think donairs are what people think of particularly when they think of Nova Scotia."

Ethical Eating

Participants who had moved to Kingston, Toronto, and Vancouver praised the expanded availability of local fresh produce, especially in Vancouver, where the growing season is longer than elsewhere in Canada. Brenda Voisey had discarded her freezer because fresh produce was accessible year-round at numerous shops near her home. In Kingston, proximity to the large agricultural area in Prince Edward County meant that fresh produce was readily available at farmers' markets or straight off the truck. It was not always clear whether this appreciation for fresh local produce sprang from an interest in health, quality, or ethics.

Regardless, those who had moved to Kingston and Vancouver also emphasized the ease with which they could engage in dominant modes of ethical eating. As we saw in Chapter 2, some Kingston families were able to buy almost exclusively local organic meat, dairy, and produce. Kristi Keller (thirty-nine, white, working poor/impoverished) commented, "At the farmers' market, you get things that are grown locally, you meet the farmers ... and you can ask 'What did you use [to grow this]? What's in your soil?' and there are organic markets – it's just a completely different way of shopping."

Ethical eating was most underscored by those who had moved to Vancouver. Brenda Voisey noted that she could get organic food almost anywhere in town. Having left Toronto eighteen years earlier, Bernice Valverde (forty-three, white, upper middle class) said that the availability of organic and ethical food was far superior in Vancouver. Keeping in mind that Toronto may have changed significantly over time, she still characterized Vancouver as a city distinctly focused on ethics:

> When I left Toronto, the first big organic food store had just opened ... The whole sort of fixation that we have with food these days was just starting to happen, I guess in the early eighties. And then being out here, a lot of our friends were involved in food production ... We had lots of people who were sort of interested in going back to the land and growing food, and we had gardens and, and I think definitely being out here changes the way in which you eat. The way in which you see food. And I'd say that the food is healthier out here.

Bernice characterized Vancouverites as simply "more interested in food," particularly in organic and sustainable food production.

The two Toronto families did not focus on ethical eating: Trudy Patterson was concerned about the cost of organic food, and Trent and Tina Payne were very involved with the connoisseur approach to cosmopolitan eating, with its stress on quality, authenticity, and rarity. The Edmonton family was deterred by the price of organic food and doubtful of the claims made for it: "When they do the tests on stuff that's supposed to be organic, it's no different from the stuff that isn't. Just more expensive" (Adam Edward, thirty-seven, white, upper middle class).

Netty Howell's Chapter 6 case study revealed that, in Halifax, it is certainly possible to be highly engaged with ethical eating. However, the Horne family, which had migrated to Halifax from Toronto, found it a challenge. When Norma Horne (forty-five, white, lower middle class) left Toronto thirteen years earlier, she was a vegetarian who ate primarily organic food. Finding this too expensive to sustain in Halifax, she returned to eating meat:

> When I moved out here, it's so much more expensive to eat well as a vegetarian that I almost immediately switched back to eating meat because it just seemed like it was economically smarter ... Some of my friends are really into the whole organic thing. And I do it to the extent that I can afford and that it's convenient.

Norma sometimes felt shamed when she had visitors from Toronto, friends who ate exclusively vegetarian and organic; she said of her inconsistent engagement with ethical eating, "I do feel guilty about it."

Healthy Eating

Ethical and healthy eating were not always clearly delineated; interviewees referred to ethical eating and health simultaneously. Urban eating was nonetheless depicted as healthy. Belinda Veitch (forty-nine, Scottish and First Nations, working poor/impoverished) and her fiancé, Bruce Vincent (forty-five, First Nations, working class), agreed that Vancouverites were healthy eaters but also noted significant dissimilarities in the city. In their mixed-income area, poorer families rented or lived in subsidized housing, whereas young, "hip" families bought relatively affordable homes and patronized the local health food stores and food co-ops. Belinda and Bruce argued that individuals who live in poverty, including most First Nations people, consume highly processed foods and plenty of salt, sugar, and fat. In contrast, Belinda saw the non-Native, more affluent members of her community as very health-focused:

> When you're talking about First Nations people in this area, their diets are horrible, really, really bad. Unless they have been told by their doctors that they have got diabetes and they got to change everything and this is what they've got to do. And if you're talking about the non-Native population in this area,

they're very health conscious. Most of them are very health conscious. They're very into organic foods.

So, though participants tended to depict Kingston, Toronto, and Vancouver (and to a lesser extent, Edmonton) as catering to ethical, cosmopolitan, and healthy eating, Belinda and Bruce warned that access to the "huge variety and excellent food" was income-dependent. In contrast, as we saw in Trudy Patterson's case study, Halifax was commonly associated with relatively unhealthy food habits. Norma Horne (forty-five, white, lower middle class) echoed Trudy's view of Halifax: "A lot of things when I first moved here just shocked me. I couldn't comprehend the whole idea of fried bologna for breakfast! It just blew me away *[laughs]*."

DEPICTING RURAL FOODWAYS

Among those who had moved to rural areas, expense and availability were significant concerns. Although she lived in Athabasca County, Annmarie Abbott (forty-five, Irish and Scottish, lower middle class) did most of her shopping in Edmonton, about two hours away. Beryl Fredericks (thirty-eight, white, lower middle class) discussed the challenges of shopping in the District of Kent, British Columbia: "We have one supermarket here and it's pretty limited in choice and it tends to be quite expensive ... So I usually shop in Chilliwack, like most people ... I don't want to pay five dollars for a jug of milk." Bette Falcon (thirty-three, Cree and French Canadian, lower middle class) lamented that though the BC Fraser Valley produces huge quantities of fruit and vegetables, most are exported, leaving locals with little access. When she lived in Vancouver, she had better access to fresh BC produce.

Pastoral Abundance and Self-Sufficiency

Most interviewees who had moved to the country depicted rural stores as having limited choice but an abundance of fresh, local produce. They also spoke positively about having the space to grow their own food. As we saw above, Karine Clements and her family grew much of their own food in Prince Edward County. After living in Yellowknife, Nina Wilkinson (forty-seven, white, upper middle class) appreciated the longer growing season in Nova Scotia's Annapolis Valley (Kings County):

> We started off last winter with fifty pounds of blueberries in our freezer. And we just bought a new chest freezer because we want to have more berries this year ... Yeah, more fruits and vegetables around, just because they're so much more abundant here ... You can get so much of it at the markets for a fairly reasonable price.

Nina and her husband also grew a wide range of vegetables in their yard. Several participants commented that almost everyone in the Annapolis Valley had a garden.

Naomi Williamson (forty-two, white, working class) thought that locally grown produce was far more available in the Annapolis Valley than it had been in her hometown of Kingston, with far more variety. She thought the cost was similar but the quality superior, and it was more readily accessible from independent producers:

> You've got more independent farmers that you can just walk up to the door and say, "Hey, can I get some goat's cheese?" Where in Ontario, you'd have to really know somebody before you could get that. It might have to be a friend of the family, or you might have to know where that farm is and hunt it down a little more. 'Cause there were farms around there, too, but it was more commercial. Here it's more hometown.

Naomi also described eating in the Annapolis Valley as "just more country style, more natural, more home-cooked. And that's what I'm trying to go toward too." She and others praised the availability of fresh fish in Nova Scotia, though acquiring it demanded some insider knowledge of where to get it from fishers – if they happened to be there. Others frequented a local lobster pound.

Though she had grown up all over Ontario and now lived in Prince Edward County, Kathleen Colbourne (forty-two, white, working poor/impoverished) had also spent time with her father "down east" in Nova Scotia. She characterized eating fish as "going back to my roots" and described learning to eat it raw while fishing with her father, who also introduced her to wild foods:

> My dad's from down east, and I spend a lot of time doing clam digging and stuff, and I love seafood ... He introduced us to all this kind of stuff ... My father tried one time to serve me snake ... I tried eel one time; I caught one in the bay ... It was, like, five, six years ago ... When I was a kid, I ate groundhog; my dad caught a groundhog and we made groundhog patties. I've tried beaver tail, I've tried wild bear ... We had to do what we had to do to survive. My father loved to hunt and fish; that's the way he was. I loved groundhog. Today, if I could get somebody to kill a groundhog – I love it.

Kathleen was Aboriginal on her mother's side, but her affinity for wild foods came from her father, who was of French and Irish heritage. Her stories construct a regional food identity, characterizing Atlantic Canada (down east) as a place of seafood, wild game, and self-sufficiency.

Like those who relocated to rural Nova Scotia, migrants to rural Prince Edward County emphasized the availability of local, fresh products. Kenzie Chambers (forty-eight, white, working poor/impoverished) had moved from Toronto three years earlier and loved knowing the people who ran small local farm markets: "There is a little stand down the road, across the road from County Traders, and their farm is all behind there, and they are only there in the summer." Kenzie spoke of buying local vegetables and beef, and mentioned that the asparagus farm was a favourite. She and her partner often fished in a nearby lake. Kendall Church (forty-one, white, working class) had moved to Prince Edward County from Montreal decades earlier. She also described the availability of fresh produce at local markets and roadside stands, and knew a number of farmers from whom she bought meat and poultry.

Similarly, in Athabasca County, Annmarie Abbott (forty-five, Irish and Scottish Canadian, lower middle class) thoroughly enjoyed local Alberta beef, which was much less available in Victoria, where she was raised. In Athabasca, she grew produce in her garden, frequented local U-pick farms to make preserves and pickles, and bought produce from a local Hutterite farm. Annette Adams (forty-three, Scottish

Canadian, upper middle class) spoke with admiration about the extent to which locals were connected to food, including the less appealing aspects of its production, compared with the more sanitized world of urbanites:

> Here people are more connected to food. If it's something that will grow in their own gardens, they'll grow it. They're actually farmers ... They butcher the chickens ... They eat meat and they understand where it comes from, and they're connected to it. They're the ones who are actively killing the animals to eat it ... To me, it seems they're more true to themselves, they're part of the whole process. [More] than people who eat meat, but it has to come in a Styrofoam container with a plastic wrapper on it and no skin on it, you know? *[laughs]*.

Likewise, Beryl Fredericks (thirty-eight, white, lower middle class) described the predominantly Dutch-heritage farmers in the Fraser Valley as having rather narrow food repertoires but suggested that "a lot of it has to do with what's available to eat. If you raise cows, you're going to eat beef. If you have a big garden, you're going to eat what you plant, and you're going to can those things. A lot of people here can be almost self-sustaining."

In Edmonton, Adam Edward (thirty-seven, white, upper middle class) described the foodways he had left behind in small-town Saskatchewan, where everyone had gardens and root cellars. He fondly recalled the emphasis on home cooking: "In Saskatchewan, there's lots of rural sons and daughters that grew up, they've watched their parents do that [cooking] by hand, all their life, so that's what they do ... 'Why would I want to go get store-bought when I can make fresh? This is way better.' And it's right."

Migrants in all the rural areas greatly appreciated the availability of fresh, local food. They valued the intimate connections to independent producers, the emphasis on homegrown and homemade, the potential for wild foods, and the pragmatic authenticity of food production. Their depictions of rural foodways emphasized pastoral purity, self-sufficiency, and genuineness. Some also suggested that social connections involving food differed in rural places. Karla Cleveland (forty-two, white, upper middle class) thought that Prince Edward

County families ate more sit-down meals than those in Toronto. Naomi Williamson (forty-two, white, working class) thought that food was more community-oriented in the Annapolis Valley: "If you look at the social board up at the mall, all you see is strawberry socials and suppers going on."

Conservative, Traditional, and Bland

Migrants often described the foodways of rural districts as conservative and rather traditional, and many sorely missed the diverse ethnic cuisines in cities. Karla Cleveland, for example, was a pragmatic cosmopolitan eater (Chapter 3), having learned to enjoy ethnic cuisines during her years in Toronto: "From being in the city and working in the city, and meeting a lot of people from different ethnicities, I love different ethnic foods!" Lacking such access in Prince Edward County, she satisfied her adventurousness through cooking:

> I'll try different things – like, I have a Thai cookbook and I remember once I made this meal, it took me an entire day, but I made all this Thai food because I wanted Thai that day *[laughs]*. I cooked everything from scratch. And it took me three or four days ahead of time to find lemon grass and all the things I needed 'cause I'd never cooked Thai before. I'm pretty adventurous!

Kristal Chirnian (forty-two, white, upper middle class) had returned to Prince Edward County after spending years in Toronto and on the West Coast. She depicted local foodways as limited and unappealing: "Food was bland and boring and represented not knowing anything better! ... Traditional meat-and-potatoes." She articulated a division between locals who had been in the County for generations and those who had moved in from elsewhere. She saw the latter as more educated, well travelled, and interested in food in a rather connoisseur cosmopolitan way. They sought out high-quality, organic, artisanal foods and loved to share food, recipes, and stories about food. Kristal saw this approach as typical among "people who are educated and who enjoy food and who have travelled and who have a life outside of the County." She added, "I hope that doesn't sound pretentious, but I think it's a reality. If you grow up in the County, it's not common. But if you have been around and you have developed other tastes, then there is a value placed on those things." In her view, long-term locals frequented diners where "you would eat meatloaf and potatoes, and you would have a bacon, lettuce, and tomato sandwich ... hot open-faced turkey sandwich, mom's meatloaf, chicken ... fish and chips, for sure."

Kendall Church (forty-one, white, working class) also mentioned a division between locals and migrants: "There's the diversity in culture and culinary food that I don't think people have been exposed to. If they're from the County, born and raised in the County, they haven't been exposed to all of the different foods ... what I was used to ... I grew up on that, more diverse food." There is definitely a sense here that education and urban environments aided in the development of a sophisticated palate.

Trent Payne (fifty-three, white, upper middle class) had grown up in a small town two hours from Toronto, surrounded by farmland. He revelled in Toronto's cosmopolitan eating and its ready access to quality restaurants, and was scathing about the food practices of his hometown:

> I am totally escaping my ethno-cultural background. I grew up in a small lunch-bucket town in Ontario, and all we ate was bologna sandwiches with ketchup *[laughs]*. That's the honest-to-God truth ... It was brutal! And my mom cooked the bejesus out of protein, boiled the snot out of Brussels sprouts. Everything was mushy vegetables and burnt beef *[laughs]*. It was terrible! ... Salads with a base of Jell-O. It was amazing *[laughs]* ... You were lucky if you had lettuce and fruit in a meal. There were tuber foods and dried protein ... Actually, when I look back on it, it was pretty abysmal.

Trent appears to be distancing himself from the food practices (and social class) of his Ontario childhood, and though his portrayal may no longer be current, he clearly associates rural eating with unhealthiness and a lack of quality, diversity, and sophistication.

The sense of a division between locals and migrants was echoed in Athabasca County, where Annette Adams described local ways of eating as "very much kind of a nondescript middle American." She added, "I hate to be critical, but food is not the focus" for locals. She stated that locals were "very limited as far as their ethnic choices on food ... The exotic thing, obviously, would be Ukrainian food." Annmarie Abbott also named Ukrainian food as the locally available "ethnic cuisine."

The absence of "ethnic restaurants" was the most common complaint of migrants in all rural areas. Bette Falcon suggested that locals in her Fraser Valley community were content with their sole Chinese restaurant and the few "ethnic" menu items at diners and family eateries "only because there's nothing else here."

Rural Nova Scotia was strongly depicted as lacking cosmopolitan food options. Natalia Warshawski (forty-seven, white, lower middle class) wondered whether "ethnic restaurants" would survive locally: "I'd like more Thai and some of the Middle Eastern food, but I don't know how they would actually survive in the area here." Nina Wilkinson (forty-seven, white, upper middle class) and Naomi Williamson (forty-two, white, working class) both characterized local eating as traditional and somewhat down to earth, though they rather enjoyed this. Nina described it as "more the Canada Food Guide kind of thing," saying, "You find still a lot of meat-eaters and just generally lots of vegetables and fruits." Similarly, Naomi described local foodways as "country-style," and she emphasized that many migrants to the Annapolis Valley held on to foodways "from away," critiquing the local manner of eating.

A comment from Nicolas Warshawski (forty-five, white, lower middle class), which presents local foodways as boring and bland, illustrates this attitude:

> Locally speaking, food is typically much less spicier. There are a few people here and there who like spicy, but on the whole not as a region have I seen a lot of people who like or adore spicy food. And Ontario is the opposite. You know, hot and spicy ... [Here] I think the food is very, very much the same ... Even pizza here, the sauces are very bland ... Even some of the spicy Chinese food here, it's not that spicy.

Nicolas's wife, Natalia, noted that "different" foods were not available in the local supermarkets, though she thought this had changed somewhat since their arrival nine years earlier: "When I first came here ... I was going to make chili and I needed white kidney beans or black beans or romano beans ... All I could find was pork and beans ... I just thought, 'How reflective of the Valley area!'"

Nigel and Nanette Wood (forty-five and forty-three, white, upper middle class) similarly characterized the foodways of rural Nova Scotia as dull, bland, and lacking in both variety and quality. Nigel suggested that "traditional" eating was taken to an extreme:

> I told Nanette when she first moved here ... She went to the local store to get matzo ball soup mix, and they didn't have it. She came back and said, "There's no matzo ball soup mix. They don't even carry it, I asked them." I said, "Nanette, if they didn't eat it in sixteenth-century England, you can't buy it here. Eat your roast beef and vegetables and potatoes and be quiet."

Nigel spoke with amusement about an incident in which Nanette, who could not find curry powder, asked the grocery clerk for help, only to learn that he had no idea what curry powder was. Nigel claimed that locals used only salt and pepper as spices. Nanette added, "some garlic salt and maybe some oregano," describing this as retrograde: "It's like what my mom made in the seventies." Nigel characterized local food-ways as backward: "It's most important to have an appreciation of food and not be stuck in this 'I must eat my cheeseburger exactly the way everyone ever has.' It just annoys me. It's like never moving out of your hometown. It's like living in your parents' basement."

Nigel and Nanette also depicted locals as poor cooks. Nigel stated,

> It's all, like, roast beef but overcooked. And then, squash – what they do to the poor squash here! I like squash if it's done right. I can barbeque a mean squash, and it turns out nicely with some brown sugar or some honey, something like that on it. But what they do is they peel the squash and they boil it 'til it's good and dead, and they mash it and add perhaps some salt and pepper just to spice it up.

The negative portrayal of Nova Scotian eating extended to Halifax. As we have seen, Norma Horne (forty-five, white, lower middle class) described the city as lacking culinary ethnic diversity, and she echoed interviewees who had moved to the Annapolis Valley: "I think Nova

Scotians tend to eat very bland food. They eat a lot of seafood, but they don't really value seafood here." Interestingly, this last comment echoes Karine Clements's statement that locals in Prince Edward County produce "artisanal-type" food but "don't even realize how special it really is." There is a similar sentiment that authentic high-quality food is wasted on locals.

Unhealthy Eating

Lastly, some participants who had migrated from the city described the foodways of their new rural areas as less healthy. In Nova Scotia, Nelda Webster (fifty-nine, white, lower middle class) thought that locals placed less importance on meals and particularly on healthy eating. More pointedly, when Karin Comeau (forty-five, white, working class) moved from Toronto to a small town in Prince Edward County, she was horrified by its eating habits, linking unhealthy diet with obesity and rurality (see McPhail, Chapman, and Beagan 2013):

> When I first moved here, I think there was five chip trucks in town. And I was appalled that this small town could keep five chip trucks alive. And, this is a staple, eating from the chip truck is just, that's just what you do, and it's cheaper ... I would watch the people go to the chip truck and watch them leave or waddle away, and I just thought, "That's so unhealthy!"

Annmarie Abbott also saw the food habits of Athabasca County farmers as unhealthy, seemingly in contrast to those of townspeople and urban migrants:

> You've got your city people in town, your town people, and then you've got your farmers. Well, I've seen farmers, that – oh man, I just wonder about their kids! Like, do they even get a meal? When I see what they're eating! A big bag of this and a big bag of that. Like, yeah to a point, sure, go ahead and have a bag of chips. But, you know, you don't need that big bag of chips.

In the case study above, Karine Clements hinted at the same thing when she said that Prince Edward County locals "shop for quantity, and so they eat more of stuff, but it's not good stuff."

CONCLUSION

As this chapter reveals, participants used discourses of healthy, ethical, and cosmopolitan eating to construct both geographic places and their own social identities. Their characterizations reflected the theoretical tension we introduced earlier, between rural spaces as idyllic and authentic, and as backward and mired in tradition (McPhail, Chapman, and Beagan 2013). Rural people themselves were portrayed as uninformed when it came to healthy, ethical, and cosmopolitan eating, unable to make the right food choices (Everett 2009). In contrast, urban foodways were generally framed positively. People in Vancouver, Toronto, Kingston, and to a lesser extent Edmonton were depicted as ethically enlightened and adventurous. Urbanites were perceived as health conscious, at least those who could afford to be.

Clearly, participants used dominant discourses of healthy, ethical, and cosmopolitan eating to mark place-related social distinctions and identities. They employed hierarchically organized symbolic capital to establish the superiority of urban Canadians (the dominant group), while simultaneously designating the practices of rural people as inferior. Some criticisms were remarkably scathing.

Interestingly, the only *regional* distinctions that stood out in our data were associated with foodways in Halifax and (to a lesser extent) Edmonton, where the negative rural image applied. For example, Halifax foodways were seen as resembling those of the Annapolis Valley – conservative, bland, and unsophisticated – and both places were constructed as uneducated and resisting modernity. Despite the fact that Halifax is a bigger city than Kingston, even when interviewees spoke positively about Halifax, their comments resembled those used to characterize rural places.

If we understand that the foodways of a place have their own logic of practice (Bourdieu 1984), rather than merely lacking the logic operating elsewhere, we are required to look at local context. Although the portrayal of Nova Scotia foodways as traditional can be seen as stereotyping, it may also contain an element of truth: The roots of many Atlantic Canadians span several generations, and community and family history in relation to place is prized. Locals joke that several generations must pass before one can legitimately claim to be "from" a place. Such a culture can foster a logic in which tradition is valued. It is the imposition of a logic from elsewhere that diminishes and casts tradition as inferior.

Although rural-urban differences seemed much clearer than regional differences, the fact that both Edmonton and Halifax had ambiguous or marginalized status in the depictions of urban foodways nonetheless suggests that the notions of core and periphery (McGillivray 2010) may still shape understandings to some extent. Vancouver, however, may have left the periphery. On the other hand, over-interpreting regional distinctions is risky here: only one Edmonton family and three from Halifax were included in the analysis for this chapter. Whereas participants who moved to Kingston, Toronto, and Vancouver typically came from smaller places, those who relocated to Halifax had lived in much larger centres. Remember that one interviewee who had moved to Edmonton from small-town Saskatchewan found its food practices sophisticated and cosmopolitan, whereas two who had left Edmonton for Vancouver depicted its foodways as narrow and conservative.

Thus, people who migrate within Canada can characterize local food practices to "make distinctions from each other that are real in their consequences, as they embody ways to differentiate themselves from those whom they denigrate" (Pugh 2011, 3). The symbolic capital of dominant groups – urbanites and possibly those outside Atlantic Canada and the Prairies – can be used to draw hierarchical boundaries of inclusion and exclusion. Such boundaries can cast "inferior" groups as lacking in taste, intelligence, and virtue (Lawler 2005). In these ways, discourses of healthy, ethical, and cosmopolitan eating can be used to characterize places and social identities, simultaneously drawing on and reinscribing particular constructions of regions and rural-urban places.

8

movement
to canada

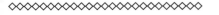

The Edo-Khel Family

THE EDO-KHEL FAMILY arrived in Canada from Pakistan four years ago. They have three children – a young son, Adil (seven), and two daughters, Atifa (fourteen) and Anwar (thirteen). Both Armin (forty-six) and his wife, Aliya (thirty-seven), hold graduate degrees. Aliya works at a preschool/ daycare centre, and Armin was unemployed when the study began. Their annual household income was low for Edmonton, at $37,000. During the study, Armin began working in community social services, substantially raising their earnings.

In Pakistan, the Edo-Khels were part of the upper social strata, but they face low income in Canada and must accept jobs that reflect neither their skills nor their qualifications, as Canadian employers do not recognize their credentials and work experience. Aliya commented on the change in status: "It's hard. Like, you have a very good status over there, and when you move here, you have nothing. It's like starting over again."

For the Edo-Khels, cooking Pakistani food is a crucial means of maintaining cultural traditions and a sense of identity, as well as transmitting their heritage and values to their children. Despite preparing it on a daily basis, Aliya also likes to experiment with new foods and cuisines, relying on both cookbooks and friends to acquire recipes. The children's tastes have been changing since the family arrived in Alberta, resulting in more work for Aliya as she attempts to accommodate their preference for more Western foods: "Especially my youngest daughter, she doesn't like our [Pakistani] food most of the time. She doesn't like to eat curry. She doesn't like to eat vegetables. So if I'm making these things, then I have to make macaronis or chicken for her. My son, he likes vegetables, so he's okay. But my daughters, they're a little bit different." Armin attributed his daughter's resistance to Pakistani food as youthful rebellion.

Cultural traditions also shape food practices when one entertains guests. Armin states that a host must always offer food, whatever the time or reason for a visit: "Offer food to anyone, even if the whole household is without food, hungry, right? You have to offer food to a guest coming to your home." Certain customs must be followed: the host must insist that everyone partake and should stop eating when guests do: "When guest stops, then everyone stops; host not supposed to take anything unless plates of everyone full." A guest must partake of everything, regardless of his or her preferences. Aliya recalls visiting a friend and disliking the food but says, "I couldn't throw out in front of her. I ate it but I didn't like it."

Food is also an important component of the Edo-Khels' religious practices. As Muslims, they require halal foods, especially meats, prepared in particular ways. Because halal foods are not easy to obtain in Edmonton, the family eats at home most of the time. Following religious dietary proscriptions can be difficult, and the Edo-Khels sometimes identify as vegetarian to avoid non-halal meat. Lack of control over ingredients or uncertainty about what a dish contains mean that dining out is a challenge.

As is common in South Asian households, Aliya – the mother – is the primary cook: "My husband, he doesn't know how to cook, so I'm the only one who cooks. My daughters, they don't know how to cook." Aliya works either a morning shift from 7:00 a.m. to mid-afternoon or an afternoon shift from mid-morning to 6:00 p.m. She budgets her time to feed her family:

> If I'm on my early shift, I come home early so I can prepare at that time too. Or sometimes what I do is when we're done eating, like, we do our supper, and then after that I cook for the next day. So the next day when I come, or the children come, there is something for them for the supper. And when we have our supper, after that I cook for the next day. And when I go on

day shift, so I'm trying to cook early in the morning, like, I usually wake up at 6:30 that time, so I cook something in the morning then.

Occasionally, Aliya will cook extra on weekends "because if I come home from my job and I'm too much tired, I don't want to cook, so sometimes I make and put it in the freezer and then just take it out." She does not use this strategy often, because she and her family prefer the taste of fresh food.

Aliya enjoys cooking for the family and is proud of being good at it. She recalls a bit of tension as a newlywed when she began learning how to cook: "Sometimes my mother-in-law, she would say, 'She's not cooking very good' [laughs]. Yeah, my sister-in-law, she would say, 'She's not cooking very good.' But I didn't cook before like that. Yeah, but now I'm a very good cook [laughs]." In most of South Asia, it is customary for a bride to live with her husband's family, which can be a source of stress for a young woman as she tries to learn the ways of her new kin, including food preferences. Nevertheless, living with an extended family meant that there were people around to help, in contrast to life in Canada, where the busy Edo-Khels are on their own. In Canada, however, Armin often helps with the dishes, and he and Aliya commonly do the food shopping together.

In Muslim Pakistan, men typically eat before women do. Neither the Edo-Khels nor Aliya's family of origin follow this practice. As Aliya explains, "It's a tradition over there. Men eat first, then women. Yeah. But for us it's not ... [And in my family] my father said, 'No, I'll start lunch at the same time.' So they ate separately in different areas, but he started at the same time." Thus, Armin and Aliya challenge traditional gender norms concerning foodwork and consumption.

Overall, the Edo-Khels deal with issues that are typical for immigrant families, of struggling to reproduce traditions while adapting to changed circumstances such as lower socio-economic status, diminished availability of customary foods, and time restrictions. This family exemplifies the complexity of everyday life; people do not merely reproduce gender norms but act in ways that reflect family and individual beliefs and practices. Similarly, food practices are not simply hierarchical, reflecting age and gender patterns, but also vary by family and individual, as seen with Aliya and Armin's renegotiation of kitchen space/foodwork and willingness to accommodate their children's tastes.

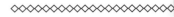

THIS CHAPTER EXPLORES how migration to Canada affects food practices and how migrants use food to situate themselves in relation to place. Through the multi-sensorial aspects of food (involving touch, taste, smell, sight), people perform their identities and connections with others across time and space. Many scholars have documented how food connects migrants with "home," re-creating its taste in a new land (Avakian 2005; Lawton et al. 2008; Vallianatos and Raine 2008; Chapman, Ristovski-Slijepcevic, and Beagan 2011; D'Sylva and Beagan 2011). The food that makes up a person's diet, the recipes used to prepare it, and the way in which it is consumed are among the most visible symbols of ethnic identity. The preparation of food from home can be a major means of transmitting cultural practices and identities across generations. For South Asian migrants, such as the Edo-Khels, continued consumption of "Pakistani food" can be integral to maintaining connection to homeland and a sense of ethnic identity. At the same time, food may be a vehicle for the embodiment of shifting identities within migrant families, who are transnational conduits of tastes and preferences (Appadurai 1996).

For decades, research in migrant communities focused on the processes and timing of "food acculturation," assuming that people who moved to a new country or a new place would eventually adopt its foodways, relegating those of their former homeland to special occasions (see Satia-Abouta et al. 2002; Varghese and Moore-Orr 2002; Lawton et al. 2008). With changes in territorial boundary marking, global media, travel, and communication technology, movement to a new part of the world no longer assumes cultural adaptation and eventual acculturation. Rather, new transnational affiliations and identities may traverse borders to maintain ongoing deeply felt connections to multiple places and nation-states (Appadurai 1996; Das Gupta 1997; Ong 1999). People may remain attached to the tastes of "home" *and* adopt those of the new place, signifying simultaneous commitment to more than one locale (Chapman and Beagan 2013).

Eating both "traditional" and Western foods may be part of the performance of place for transnational migrants. At the same time, food practices are also shaped by global forces. The traditional foods of the old homeland may be changing even as they are fiercely retained by migrants (Collins 2008). With the movement of capital, ideas, objects, and people across borders, the neat divide between traditional and Western cuisine diminishes as food practices and items are adopted globally – in part through the movement of people across borders.

THEORETICAL FRAMING

Although globalization and movement have always been part of human history, their contemporary manifestations evoke the common perception that the world's present state of flux is unique in history. Scholars investigating experiences and perceptions of mobility in the last few decades have focused on tourism, diasporas, global markets and media, cosmopolitanism, and transnationalism. More recently, social and spatial theorists have linked embodied experiences with ideologies and meanings of mobility and immobility (or mooring), emphasizing that "the colonial world economy has long entailed extensive global mobilities – e.g. of slaves, of commodities, of print and images and of capital" (Sheller 2011, 2).

Anthropological thinking on the formation of transnational subjects (who are simultaneously attached to more than one nation, see Ong 1999) and critiques of boundedness (see Appadurai 1996; Hannerz 1996; Clifford 1997) have been central in understanding the politics of mobility. Current theories of mobility merge "the more purely 'social' concerns of sociology (inequality, power, hierarchies) with the 'spatial' concerns of geography (territory, borders, scale) and the 'cultural' concerns of anthropology and media studies (discourses, representations, schemas)" (Sheller 2011, 2), while attending to the interrelations among subjects, spaces, and meanings.

In this chapter, we examine how the food practices of participants who had emigrated to Canada illustrate their experiences of mobility, crossing various types of socio-political boundaries, including within and across nation-states. We explore the positionings of multiple, complex selves in the performance of contemporary national/global mobile citizenship and cultural production, through talk and practices concerning food. It is important to remember that mobility includes not only the movement of bodies and objects but also that of ideas and imaginations (Urry 2007). The global symbol of McDonald's golden arches signifies fast food – and more abstractly, Western capitalist individualism, efficiency, and standardization – whether or not the food chain itself even exists in a particular country.

Spatial fixity and movement co-exist in overlapping, complex ways (see Sheller and Urry 2006), always a function of historical and contemporary power relations, which shape who/what becomes mobile and when movement is restricted (Adey 2010). "Mobility capital," a term coined by Kaufmann, Bergman, and Joye (2004), refers to the unequal distribution of capacities and competencies among people, determining who can and cannot move across physical and social spaces and boundaries. Not every individual or group has the same access to either mobility or the choice of whether to move or stay (Kaufmann and Montulet 2008). Mobility, and attendant capacities and competencies that facilitate it, is shaped by power relations of gender, class, ethnicity, nationality, and other social hierarchies. At the same time, competencies valued in one place may hold differing value in a new place. All our study participants who moved to Canada had relatively high mobility capital, as they were immigrants who chose to relocate. Yet their mobility capital is more complex when contextualized within the social relations in their country of origin as well as in Canada, and when intrafamily dynamics are considered, particularly concerning gender and age.

Bodies, technologies, and cultural practices come together in the performance of "movement-space" through everyday practices (see Sheller 2004; Thrift 2004). The multi-sensory performance of place connects lived bodily experiences with mobility and grounding in physical space (see Cresswell and Merriman 2011; Lee and Ingold 2006). Senses of space and movement, experienced through the body, help us construct "emotional geographies" through which space becomes place, infused with particular meanings (Sheller and Urry 2006). Because food is a multi-sensorial object that explicitly connects cultural ideas with corporeal experiences, it is a particularly valuable tool to examine mobilities and the performance of movement-space.

PARTICIPANTS, PLACES, AND APPROACH TO ANALYSIS

Twenty-one of our participant families had migrated to Canada. Seven were from Europe, one from New Zealand, two from the United States, four from East Asia, five from South Asia, one from the Horn of Africa, and one had come from West Africa via Australia. In the past, emigrants to Canada hailed primarily from Europe, but non-European origins have increasingly dominated since the late twentieth century (particularly Asian countries). In our study, the European immigrants (and the New Zealand family) were long-time residents of Canada. The only exception was a Ukrainian woman who was married to a Nigerian; the family had lived in Australia for many years prior to moving to Canada two years ago. The family from the Horn of Africa also had European connections; the mother had lived in a Southern European country before coming to Canada. Some of the Asian migrant families were long-term residents of Canada, whereas others had arrived more recently.

The families had settled in various parts of Canada: eight each in British Columbia and Ontario, four in Alberta, and one in Nova Scotia. This distribution echoes typical Canadian patterns, as most immigrants settle in or near Vancouver, Toronto, Montreal, and increasingly Edmonton, as employment opportunities expand in Alberta, particularly in relation to the oil and natural gas industry. Influxes of immigrants alter the local foodscape, as both specialized and mainstream stores cater to more diverse needs. The size of immigrant communities in urban centres affects the kinds of foods, cooking implements, and restaurants that are available to migrants.

A TASTE OF MIGRATION

The connection to "home" through food was amply evident in the narratives of migrants to Canada. As Aliya Edo-Khel from the case study above said, "We have a special kind of rice from our area [of Pakistan] ... I'm still making, and that's the special kind of rice that I asked my mom to send." An Eritrean woman, Tabia Punnu (forty-four, working poor/impoverished), also relied on her mother to send items from home, such as spices: "My mom she send [cumin] to me and then I grind it ... It's different from Canadian cumin; back home cumin is a different taste." She later noted that the "Canadian food" she had encountered "was all tasteless. There was no taste in there." Adeela Esani (forty-one, South Asian Canadian, upper middle class) was particularly eloquent about missing the tastes of Pakistan: "You see, the things I miss the most – the food doesn't have the taste it used to have back home. Taste is not here. Flowers don't have smell. And life doesn't have happiness, the true happiness. We used to live together in a small house, but there was true happiness."

Thus, through daily food practices and attempts to re-create certain tastes, migrants perform their ethnocultural identities in efforts to transcend geographically distinct spaces. Yet living in new locales can cause imperceptible shifts in performances of self through food and taste practices. Toma Patel (forty-six, Ukrainian, lower middle class) explained that living in Australia's hot climate prior to coming to Canada changed her family's food practices, encouraging the consumption of more fresh fruit and vegetables. She also described her Nigerian husband's gradual shifts in relation to food, attributing these to mobility:

> My husband changed his food habits; growing up in Nigeria, he used to have very hot, spicy foods. Since we got married, his food habits changed. Now he's gone back to his country to visit; it takes time for him to eat that food again ... Any person who moving countries, they would eventually change their habits. Mainly because there is another reason to eat [differently]. Living in Australia, he couldn't actually find his African food shops where he can buy the special different spices. And this was another reason why the person can change his habits of living and cultural background and meals. He has to eat, right?

Changes in performances of self through sensory food practices do not occur uniformly in families. This is evident between partners, such as with the Patel family, where the mother is Ukrainian and the father is Nigerian. Toma Patel divulged that sometimes her husband "cooks his traditional meal, which I don't like the taste of. And basically, he's free to cook it and to, you know, use that meal. And then I have to cook for myself as well because I'm hungry." The Patel family generally ate most meals together, with the odd exception when the father cooked Nigerian dishes. Though all the Patels had been influenced by their time in Australia, Toma tended to cook from her Ukrainian heritage and did not accommodate the preferences of her husband.

More typically, women learned to oblige their husband's tastes after marriage. Adeela Esani and her in-laws came from different parts of India, and she was expected to learn their foodways:

I had to learn from my in-laws their types of cooking, 'cause when
I was there, they want me to help in their meal; they don't want to
eat what I know how to cook. So initially, I had to cook whatever
my husband used to eat, like what my mother-in-law cooked. So I
had to learn her type of cooking.

Divergent food preferences can be a source of friction, particularly
between generations. As we saw in Chapter 5, Adeela Esani constantly
struggled with her children, especially her eldest son, Aarya, about the
consumption of Pakistani dishes. Her children identified with "brown
food," seeing it as part of their cultural heritage, yet simultaneously
resisted Pakistani foods (and ideals), preferring "Canadian" foods and
food practices. Aarya's opposition was marked by his preference for
eating out with friends. Arjan, the younger son, exhibited less overt
resistance but preferred Western food for both meals and snacks.

These experiences of shifting tastes are echoed in the exchanges
between children in another family. Abeer Ebrahim (fourteen, Pakistani Canadian, upper middle class) and her brother Ahsan (ten)
migrated from Pakistan six years ago. Asked why they liked to eat
Pakistani food, Abeer said, "Since we're used to it, we think that it's,
like, better food than what people usually eat over here." Nonetheless,
she and Ahsan acknowledged that their tastes were changing:

ABEER: In Pakistan, we used to have Pakistani foods every day
and all the time. Over here, there's fast-food restaurants
and, like, pizza. In Pakistan, there was still, like, Pizza
Hut and things like that, but we didn't really like pizza
over there, and we like it over here.

AHSAN: I think I liked it both places, but I'm used to here. But I
want to go to Pakistan again and try their food again.

In South Asia, eating at fast-food restaurants like Pizza Hut is
typically a treat or a marker of high social status. Chains generally
modify their menus to suit local tastes, so the comments of Abeer
and Ahsan are interesting in their preference for "Canadian" foods in
Canada. Furthermore, Ahsan's reflections emphasize his socialized
sensory experiences – "I'm used to here." He wants to test his perception of difference by tasting pizza in Pakistan again.

When children resist traditional foods, this may underscore age-based divergences in ethnocultural identities and performances. Kavitha Kirmani (forty-seven, South Asian Canadian, upper middle class) described how her son, Kumar (sixteen), has "had a bit more North American influence, so therefore, you know, *[whining]* 'I don't wanna eat this.' He eats it anyway, 'cause I make him." Children's resistance to traditional foods, or even preference for Western ones, can be interpreted as a rejection of family and ethnocultural heritage. Plus, as we saw in the Edo-Khel case study, it creates more work for mothers, who typically cook for the family. As Aliya Edo-Khel noted, "If I'm making something that's especially from our culture, then I have to make something else for them too." Adeela Esani echoed, "Back home when we had parties, only traditional dishes [were served]. But here, some children are coming, and they've only lived in Canada. So they don't like those curries."

On the other hand, children may bring "tastes of Canada" to older family members through foods not typically consumed in their countries of origin, such as pasta and salads. Although some families adopt these foods, the tensions of transnationalism are ever-present. For example, the Esani children emphasized that they liked pasta; as Aarya (twenty) said, "We'll make curry and stuff, but we'll make pasta on the side." Yet his mother, Adeela, stated that her husband refuses to eat pasta: "I just can't have spaghetti or lasagna. My husband won't eat that. He'll never eat that. He has never tried lasagna, although I've cooked it so many times. He says he just cannot have it. He's never tried it or pasta. Even if I cook it, I have to cook something else for my husband."

New tastes can embody tensions of mobility within families, as the unfamiliar is corporeally experienced. But even most migrant adults noted sensory shifts over time, creating potential conflicts within themselves in terms of identity and place. As Barjinder Virk (fifty-seven, South Asian Canadian, working class) stated during a discussion of food types and styles, "We are very uncomfortable with mushrooms." But then, to signal her and her family's adjustment in a new space, she said, "Brussels sprouts, this kind of vegetable we always have it. Asparagus we like." Choosing to highlight two vegetables that are often associated with special meals and that have strong tastes (particularly Brussels sprouts) suggests that Barjinder is performing comfort with a new space through knowledge of items that are not part of South Asian cuisines. Furthermore, Brussels sprouts in particular are often badly cooked and strong tasting, and are usually an acquired taste in North America. Because asparagus can be expensive (as its growing season is short), consuming it can be a sign of social status, and knowledge of certain foods and their preparation can indicate local cultural expertise.

Performances of such food knowledge can lessen gaps between distant and current physical spaces, though they can also highlight distance. Interestingly, asparagus also featured in Adele Eichmann's (forty-six, German Canadian, lower middle class) yearnings, as she discussed German cookbooks and cooking styles: "That's asparagus ... It's just a little booklet [on cooking asparagus]. Because where I'm from, they plant a lot of asparagus. Oh, I miss that! The white asparagus. There was a white asparagus, you know; it's tiny, yeah."

Many migrants strategically incorporated certain Canadian foods into their culinary repertoire, not only for ease of preparation and because they appealed to children (such as pasta), but also for health. Such was the case for Torma Pala (forty, Tibetan Canadian, lower middle class), who favoured retaining traditional ethnocultural food in her family's diet but was nonetheless open to "healthy" Canadian examples: "Tibetan food, like, some of the foods it's very important really. As we are Tibetan, we should have that food ... How important our language is, that's how important that food is also." Yet she added, "Other food, even Canadian food [if they] are better, why don't we try those ones?" Torma explained the importance of Tibetan food for her family's identity and noted that she wanted her daughter, Tashi (fifteen), to include it in her diet. Even so, she was open to other food, as long as it was healthy: "Whatever she make, healthy food, whatever she cook at home, that's very important. If it's healthy, whether it's Canadian, Indian, Tibetan, whatever." In contrast, many migrants associated a "taste of Canada" with sugar and fat, as Bao Vai (forty-one, Chinese Canadian, working class) did in discussing the preferences of her daughter Bernie (fourteen): "She likes sweet things. I think that's for most Canadians, right? You like the sweet things *[laughs]*. And deep-fry *[laughs]*."

Lastly, the tastes of migration are not unidirectional. Although parents may attempt to teach their children the tastes of home, and children may resist traditional foods, migrants may also bring tastes in multiple directions across borders by introducing Western cuisines to their families. The Patels, a family of Ukrainian and Nigerian origin, attributed their preference for particular kinds of salads to time spent in Australia. Adeela Esani explained that she shared Canadian-acquired tastes during family visits to Pakistan: "From Canada to Pakistan, we take cookies and chocolate and nuts. When I was in Pakistan last year, we took cereal. My kids like certain kinds of cereal, and we don't have lots of variety there, just corn flakes, that's it. So my children like Cheerios, so we took that. And cookies and chocolate." When the interviewer asked, "Your extended family likes that stuff?" she replied, "For sure."

This illustrates the complexity of global migration experiences; no longer unidirectional flows from one place to another, as was common in the past, they are multidirectional in varying degrees, as technologies (such as air travel and social media) allow a more frequent traversing of boundaries and places. However, such passages are moderated by social class and values, as a family's financial status affects its access to technologies and the means to traverse space, and their social values shape how such resources are used. For example, migrants to Canada commonly have limited financial resources. Despite a downward shift in socio-economic status after migration, Adeela's family chose to make frequent trips to Pakistan to ensure that the children did not forget their ethnocultural identity. This still posed financial hardship, as Adeela pointed out:

> We had to spend so much money! But we had to go. This is our seventh year in Canada, and we've visited four times. Some things are not counted with money. Money is nothing when it comes to your children's happiness and well-being. And I want them to see their culture with their own eyes instead of me telling them this is how it works back home ... My children still know how to read and write in Urdu. They speak so well, they know their culture, they're willing to get married in Pakistan. People who don't take their children back home, they don't know the language, they don't like the dress, they don't like the food, and they don't want to marry back home. So how do you keep the culture alive? It's really hard. We never came to Canada to lose our culture and values.

This family, however, was not as financially constrained as many others, who might wish to visit their homelands but simply could not afford the expense or the time off work. Changes in performances of self through sensory experiences of food are at least partly dependent on social position after migration; without the resources to travel, culinary connections to home may increasingly stray from the imagined reality.

In sum, food and the quality of taste can reveal how mobility is dependent on complex intersections of fields of power. A distant "home" is reconstructed as unchangingly tasteful, whereas unsettling movement coincides with "tasteless" food in the new locale. Disjunctions of belonging and place merge with disjunctions of taste. Yet spatial movement overlaps with spatial fixity, evident in the often imperceptible shifts in food preferences over time, as immigrants strategically adopt new food and take new tastes and foods back home. Spatial movement and fixity intersect with particular fields of power in relation to age (tensions between children and adults), gender (shifts in expectations), and social class (capacities to return home).

PREPARING AND CONSUMING FOOD AND SELF

The concept of performed movement-space – the embodied, emplaced practice of self – can be understood not only through the taste of food, but also through its preparation and consumption, which reflect social location and understanding of self. For immigrants, these aspects of food performance further highlight acceptance and belonging, or rejection and exclusion.

Food preparation is one way of performing ethnocultural identity. Betje Fortuyn (forty-eight, Dutch, working class) stated, "We eat kale not like the Canadians do" and gave a detailed explanation of how she had learned to prepare it in Holland. Bao Vai, who migrated from China fourteen years earlier, differentiated herself from other Canadians by how she cooked vegetables: "We cook it not like you; you make it like salad. You don't cook right most of the vegetables. Most of the vegetables we cook, put some oil and then put the vegetables and then steam, boil." Theo and Talia Rousseau (forty-four and forty-nine, French, upper middle class) compared food cultures in France and Canada, with Theo noting that "caring about food" was the norm in France: "Food is a big part of your day." Talia remarked that "the

French are much better about respecting" seasonal availability of food, thus affecting how one cooks.

Performance of ethnocultural identity through food preparation is gendered in particular cultural ways. In some migrant families, especially from Asia, girls were expected to acquire cooking skills, whereas boys were not. Adeela Esani explained,

> It's cultural; like, my husband doesn't know how to cook, and if he would have known at least how to cook something, it would have helped him over there [working in the oil fields]. But still, I don't regret that he doesn't know how to cook; this is the way we bring up our sons. I would want my daughter to know how to cook traditional and Canadian dishes, but not them [my sons].

She later reflected, "Yeah, the first thing we ask the daughter-in-law is if she knows how to cook. The first thing we want to know. What about other skills? Well, that will come, but what about cooking? My goodness! *[laughs].*" The gendering of food-related performances was particularly strong among the non-European families, many of whom had had servants in their countries of origin; the women now carried the burden of domestic work, including food preparation.

Cultural identity is also enacted through hosting. Betje Fortuyn (forty-eight, Dutch, working class) compared differences in expectations, noting that for social gatherings, "we put more food on the table here." She went on to say, "They do it the same way in Holland, but they put less food on the table, I guess. They think we eat more is what they always say when they come here." Aliya Edo-Khel noted that even in Pakistan her particular ethnic group is renowned for its hospitality: "We, the Pashtu-speaking people, we are very different. We are more hospitable. We cooked a lot, and we served a lot." This hospitality carries over to Canadian contexts, where multiple dishes are prepared for the main course, along with appetizers, side dishes, and desserts. Hosting a dinner party could sometimes mean that Aliya would be cooking for days in advance, performing her ethnocultural identity through food.

Toma Patel noted that Ukrainian hosts traditionally provided a great deal of food, so that no one could "leave your place without a full stomach." When hosting her first Christmas celebration in Canada, she had "so many foods that we had to invite [guests] the next day to finish it." Although Toma had retained the emphasis on quantity, she had slightly changed her approach, beginning to ask guests to bring "their best food" to share.

How one eats can also indicate ethnocultural affiliation. For instance, Betje Fortuyn noted that "most of the time we mash our potatoes" and added, "Most of the time we put them on our plate; we mash everything and then you mash everything together, and then you start eating. That's the Dutch way ... Certain meals you have to mash, otherwise they don't taste good."

Eating also includes body techniques – how one sits, holds utensils or hands, and so on. Ayesha Ebrahim (forty, Pakistani Canadian, upper middle class) stated that eating with the hands is typical in Pakistan, a practice the family continued post-migration. Tatjana Radanovic (fifty-three, Serbian Canadian, lower middle class) voiced frustration with the speed of eating in Canada. This caused tensions with her seventeen-year-old son, who ate much faster than she:

> I cannot stand when I prepare everything and he finishes first and he just leaves. I want to kill him! Sit here, slow, I want to hear about your day! Like French people are really good at – they never rush through the food, and Italians too, they take time. But here, everything is like [snaps fingers].

Theo and Talia Rousseau found it "shocking" that families did not sit together around a dinner table or put much thought and preparation into their menu.

Body techniques of eating can also include where one eats, the physical space in which food is consumed. Aliya Edo-Khel described gendered eating spaces among Pakistani migrants in her circle in Edmonton: the women typically sat in chairs around the table, and the men took their food into another room. She noted, however, that these divisions were variable even in Pakistan: "We grew up in cities, so it's different for us. But those who are only in the countryside, they have to cover their faces up here [to eyes], and they even don't allow [women] to say hello to [male visitors]." Aliya's father ate at the same time as the female members of his family, not before, but she added that the women were "not allowed to come in front of men who we don't know."

Thus, when male company was expected, Aliya would arrange every-thing in the dining room, "and then men have separate space [to eat] and the women have separate, and they don't even have to come in front [of the men]."

Consumption as identity performance can also focus on the foods that constitute meals – which may be affected by daily schedules. For example, migrants who are accustomed to eating their main meal in mid-day, as Theo Rousseau reported was the case in France, cannot re-create this in the context of the Canadian work day. Research among immigrants has shown that breakfast foods are often first to change (see Ray 2004). This is probably due to a shift in daily routines accompanying settlement in a new place, and the morning meal on weekdays may be particularly rushed. Consequently, breakfast is often the first meal that shifts in content and context. Time constraints in the morning (commutes, school bus schedules) dictate breakfast routines. Quick breakfast foods, such as cereal, may be incorporated into migrant food practices.

But as noted above, changes do not necessarily occur uniformly in a family and may vary according to age and gender. For example, mothers who do not work outside the home or are not as rushed in the morning may be able to continue traditional breakfast patterns. This diversity in families was illustrated by Barjinder Virk (fifty-seven, South Asian Canadian, working class), as she talked about her son's preferences: "In breakfast, he likes to eat cereal. Me, I like to eat the leftovers. I just like my own food. My East Indian food, right. Cauli-flower, potatoes, and curry. I like this. Sometimes I eat cereal, but I don't fond of it. My kids like to eat cereal."

Emphasizing the significance of time for food patterns, Barjinder noted that in her own family a parent was always home to prepare East Indian foods, which may take time to create. But time-saving meas-ures may also be used (buying herb packets rather than grinding). Availability of such convenience foods varies by place. Krista Kwan (fifty-two, Chinese Canadian, upper middle class) noted that at Kingston's Chinese grocery store, "we're getting more instant food but not as quick as, like, the Kraft Dinner sort of thing. We can buy packages of sauces now, all prepared for you too. And you can buy fro-zen dumplings, in Toronto." Some families infrequently made ethno-cultural foods, "just for those special things," as Adele Eichmann remarked. Torma Pala stated that, surrounded by dominant Euro-Canadian ways of eating, "nowadays many people, they are changing."

Alterations in identity performances through how and what migrants eat can reflect not only shifting allegiances, but also socio-cultural values and mores, as well as available technology. Adeela Esani argued that children in Canada don't value anything, that everything was taken for granted. In Pakistan, no one sold meat on Tuesdays and Wednesdays: "That means that Tuesdays and Wednesdays, you don't get any meat. So you end up eating vegetables and lentils." In Canada, she had a large freezer and bought meat in bulk, so it was always available: "Back home, the trend is not buying in bulk. You buy for two or three days only. So my children used to value that, Tuesdays and Wednesdays, they didn't get any meat; so then they used to value it, two days without meat and then they got it on Thursdays. When they got it then, they valued the meat." Adeela's comment suggests that the availability of technology and the social values of consumerism have diminished the meaning attached to food in her family.

The performance of movement-space is partly contingent upon access to necessary resources. The size of immigrant communities in urban centres affects the kinds of foods, cooking implements, and restaurants available, as noted by Kavitha Kirmani (forty-seven, South Asian Canadian, upper middle class), who said that a *tava* (a griddle used for cooking roti or *paranthas*) could be found in Toronto, though not Kingston. Another Kingston participant, Krista Kwan, described loading up on Chinese foodstuffs whenever she visited Toronto: "Every couple months we go to Toronto, we'll buy some Chinese groceries ... Like, we'll bring a large cooler ... At least four or five times a year. Or any time we happen to be in Toronto, we make sure we have a cooler with us."

At the same time, most participants emphasized that knowledge of North American food practices was not confined to North America, in a global economy. Aliya Edo-Khel stated that offering guests "ginger ale or Sprite or Coke or Pepsi" was a tradition "not only here but back home too." Many interviewees had experienced global foods through exposure to multinational food companies and restaurant chains. Because such food was typically expensive, knowledge of it was linked with social class, and consuming it symbolized status and cosmopolitanism. As Adeela Esani indicated, ketchup and soya sauce, which are ordinary condiments in Canada, are specialty items in Pakistan. Thus, some foods were not unfamiliar after migration, and participants had some knowledge in purchasing foods in grocery stores or in choosing places to eat out.

Finally, it is important to note that particular performances of movement-space through food are practically demanded of migrants. Armin Edo-Khel (forty-six, Pakistani, upper middle class) spoke disparagingly of the workshops and seminars aimed at non-European migrants to assist their settlement through imparting knowledge of where to shop, what to buy, and how to prepare unfamiliar items. Armin pointed out that such classes not only propagate hegemonic or dominant knowledge, but also Other migrants by assuming no familiarity with North American foods and cooking styles:

> I think this is wrong ... Canadian cooking class, what do you mean by Canadian cooking class? Why are you forcing these people to assimilate? Why are you forcing them to give their kids pasta? ... We do the pasta and hamburger, hot dogs and other stuff. That we have, the same was there [Pakistan] too ... For God's sake, they know how to cook! They know how to cook, what is healthy food, they know it. The problem is that they don't have money!

Armin contended that such workshops draw on the age-old perception of the migrant Other as a kind of savage barbarian:

> People are not coming from the jungle. This is a very wrong perception. When you see an African, quickly a thing comes to your mind: a jungle, a lion, a bear, and this is not the case. They are highly civilized people. They have a history of civilization and thousands of years of civilization. They're not coming from the jungle. But here people have this distorted, different [image].

In contrast, Armin urged migrants to perform ethnocultural identities and relationship to place and mobility though adhering to their own food practices: "Demonstrate your culture. Instead of going for Canadian cooking, do your own cooking. Tell the Canadians that this is something healthy ... Introduce those things." The complexity, of course, is that as Armin himself pointed out, the foods of "home" also include global foods; the boundaries of places are permeable in a global economy marked by transnational mobility.

CONCLUSION

Food as a material and emotive social object helps us to elucidate the complex ways in which immigrants negotiate spaces, belonging, and identity. Throughout this chapter, we have emphasized how migrant individuals, families, and communities employ food practices to perform their identities in relation to particular places. All migrant participants enjoyed high mobility capital, but they nonetheless faced disjunctions and constancies. Some attempted to hold on to the tastes of "home," some resisted the foods of home (especially youth), and some used quite specific foods (such as Brussels sprouts) to signify social belonging, or at least culinary comfort. Most participants spoke of shifting tastes and food practices, but some also noted that North American foods were prized consumables in other parts of the world. Thus, immigrants as a group concurrently embody spatial fixity and movement, but variable performances of movement-space arise from each individual's experiences and sense of identity.

Participants' embodiment of spatial fixity/movement was evident in their performances of place and identity through food preparation, hosting and being hosted, eating itself, and the use of food-related spaces. In all these dimensions, change and maintenance were complicated by age and generation. In other words, though immigrants as a group share broad experiences of spatial movement, actual lived experiences vary in ways that reflect fields of power. Immigrant parents are typically invested in passing on their traditional food practices to their children, whereas the children themselves may concentrate on fitting into their current social environment. Simultaneously, postmigration shifts in time use and access to food-related technologies and resources may create friction in families. These may have differential impact by gender, as women most commonly shoulder the task of feeding families in the face of conflicting food desires and identity performances.

$$9$$

embodiment

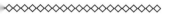

The Aronowitz Family

THE ARONOWITZ FAMILY lives on a farm in northern Alberta's Athabasca County, where oil development and associated spinoff jobs have brought a degree of prosperity. The median annual income is fairly high, at over $63,000. Agnes Aronowitz (fifty-one) is a teacher, and her husband, Alfred (fifty-three), works in the trades, with a combined income of $90,000 annually. They are white and of British and Eastern European heritage, although Agnes self-identifies as "Canadian." The Aronowitzs have two older children who are away at college and two teenage children at home: Alyssa (eighteen), who is about to leave for college, and a son, Aleksy (sixteen).

The sensorial aspects of food are of critical importance to this family, both in procurement and consumption. Taste is Agnes's top priority, and she speaks passionately about the superior flavour of homemade and homegrown food:

> It's so much better! When I made a blueberry pie out of store-bought blueberries, my family said, "What did you do to this pie? It doesn't taste

very good." Yeah, you can tell. My husband, if I buy corn from the store, he probably wouldn't eat it. If we have it off our garden, there's a huge difference in taste.

This perceived difference between store-bought and homemade is echoed in the family's preference for raising its own food – both plant and animal. For the Aronowitzs, quality is closely connected with taste.

Simple, tasty food is a way of life for them. They describe their diet as meat-and-potatoes, an eating style that is common throughout the Prairies and the Midwestern United States, and often associated with farming. They see food as central to connecting and sharing with family across generations. Sit-down family meals are the norm, and they rarely eat out at restaurants, preferring to entertain friends at home. They take pleasure in everything connected with food, though their repertoire is not adventurous or exotic. Agnes enjoys gardening, baking, and preserving, and is pleased that her family appreciates her skills. She occasionally works with her husband in the garden, which enables them to spend time together. Agnes takes pride in being recognized for her abilities: "I'm noted as the mom that cooks good."

Agnes takes her values to work, where she recently attempted to convey the sensorial aspects of good, tasty food to the small children she teaches but was hampered by safety controls:

> To have the kids, show them how to dig the carrot out of the ground, wash it, taste it, and then taste this one – there's so much more ownership here. And even, there's been some schools that have raised their own little garden. Or even going – I used to take my school kids, my classroom school kids, to a dairy farm. But I haven't done that lately 'cause there's not the accessibility any more. You can't go there 'cause you might con-taminate ... We might bring something into that barn. So I've tried to do things like that, but it doesn't work.

The Aronowitzs have a close relationship to the land, relying on home-grown and homemade foods. For them, the notion of a "local food en-vironment" is not a hundred-mile diet, but rather food that they grow, harvest, and cook. They have little interest in ethical eating, as they already raise most food themselves. Agnes laughingly recalled a discussion with her brother, who lives in an urban centre, in which he praised her carrots, saying, "'Gee, these carrots are just like farmers' market carrots!'

And I said, 'Well of course! Where do you think the farmers' market ones come from?' *[laughs]*." The Aronowitzs are quite self-sufficient in terms of food, relying not only on their own gardens, but also those of relatives. They regularly trade or share meat and fish with other family members, shopping only for staples and sundry products at grocery stores.

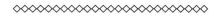

IN PREVIOUS CHAPTERS, we argued that the concept of habitus (Bourdieu 1984) is central to understanding the symbolic role of food in marking social relations. In this chapter, we explore how the habitus is formed and changed, examining how sensorial qualities of food and eating interact in specifically classed and gendered locations – in families – to create embodied experiences that inform the creation of dispositions. The chapter forefronts the body – how food becomes incorporated into our cells and souls, and how food norms and values as well as normative everyday eating practices become embedded in our sensory selves. This approach problematizes the mind-body divide, which is prevalent in Western thought and which prioritizes thought over embodied experience (Desjarlais 1992).

Academic studies of the body tend to remain predominantly theoretical, with a curious neglect of the experiential aspects of embodiment (Thomas and Ahmed 2004). This chapter helps to address this gap, by focusing on the role of the senses, particularly taste, in the process of embodiment and self-making, as well as social identity construction. It asks how people use physical sensations and experiences in understanding and expressing their ideas of who they are and their relationships with others. This self-making process, we suggest, is informed both implicitly and explicitly through sensory everyday experiences, which are themselves culturally informed.

THEORETICAL FRAMING

Western ideologies have placed the body in hierarchical opposition to the mind and seen it as inferior: more animalistic and therefore less valuable or important. Since the time of Aristotle, Western thought has hierarchized the senses, seeing taste and touch as lesser than sight and hearing, and placing smell in the middle (Vinge 2009). In this tradition, the five senses correspond with parts of the body. However, this understanding of the senses and their bodily location is a cultural construction; how bodies and senses are conceptualized varies across time and space. For example, in some cultures, body boundaries are viewed as permeable and susceptible to sensory crossings. Smell can infiltrate another body, carrying negative feelings and qualities, and can thus infect it, resulting in illness (Desjarlais 1992). Understanding divergent culturally specific ways of making sense of physical sensations is essential to cross-cultural work with pain, illness, and health (see Hay 2008; Throop 2008).

The Western approach to the senses is also gendered, as the more "animalistic" ones – touch, taste, and smell – have been associated with women. Constance Classen (2005) argues that touch, taste, and smell were viewed as nurturing, seductive, and non-bounded (they could easily cross boundaries between self and other). They needed to be properly controlled, and women's traditional roles of wife and mother were a means of setting sensory boundaries. Touch, taste, and smell connect women to others in part through foodwork. In Canada today, women still do most of the food shopping, preparation, and cleanup (Beagan et al. 2008). Mothers become important agents of imparting knowledge and values to their families via the tastes, textures, and scents conveyed through food and cooking (Seremetakis 1994). Sensory messages are unconsciously incorporated into embodied experiences of self and other, becoming part of one's habitus.

Embodied ways of being-in-the-world (the habitus), including sensory feelings, are also a classed phenomenon. From our earliest moments of socialization, our sensory milieus are linked to class-related experiences. As Bourdieu (1984, 6) suggests, the learned (yet subconscious) "taste of liberty or luxury" enjoyed by the upper classes contrasts with the "taste of necessity" internalized by the working classes. Members of the upper classes are socialized to value particular aesthetic experiences that become incorporated into bodily practices, including eating – the so-called tastes of luxury shaping how food is prepared, presented, and consumed. Bourdieu described the taste of luxury as including "light foods," which fit into a relatively sedentary lifestyle yet do not create bodily discomfort (such as a sense of fullness); following class-defined norms, they have sensorial appeal and simultaneously symbolize affluence. In contrast, the taste of necessity includes filling, heavy foods, sustaining the physical labour of the working classes. Thus, Bourdieu explicitly linked the sensation of taste with class aesthetics.

Carolyn Korsmeyer (1999) distinguished between "taste" as gustatory sensation and "Taste" as metaphorical, aesthetic, culturally constructed perceptions reflecting particular social norms and values. Yet she insisted that Bourdieu's social and class distinctions in Taste must never be understood as separate from individual sensory pleasures and aversions. Korsmeyer urged greater attention to the body in investigating how taste and Taste intertwine. This chapter builds on these ideas, exploring how sensory, embodied selves perform and experience cultural norms and values that are situated in particular instances of time and space. As we examine how sensory selves are constructed and understood, we inevitably consider how the senses are simultaneously gendered, classed, and otherwise marked.

PARTICIPANTS, PLACES, AND APPROACH TO ANALYSIS

This chapter examines data from all participants in British Columbia, Alberta, and Nova Scotia. The relevant interviews involved twenty-two mothers, six fathers, and twenty-five teens in British Columbia; twenty-one mothers, five fathers, and thirty-one teens in Alberta; and twenty mothers, four fathers, and twenty-seven teens in Nova Scotia. To analyze the data, we examined those parts of participant interviews that we had coded "body knowledge" as well as opinions and experiences related to the sensory aspects of food (coded as "taste/ smell/texture"). We also searched all interviews for any mention of "taste" or "flavour." Finally, we examined how these passages intersected with passages that we had coded as "culture/tradition," "upbringing," and "learning/teaching" to explore how sensory aspects of food were shaped by social, cultural, and familial context.

EMBODIED TASTE, EMBODIED VALUES

Because implicit learning occurs every day, the family kitchen and family table are crucial locations for embodied learning among children. This is illustrated in the Aronowitz case study, where Agnes's emphasis on taste and quality was an ongoing component of her food provisioning: "I've done that ever since day one." The impact was evident in her older children, who visited (with friends) to take advantage of their mother's fine cooking and who explicitly asked her to grow certain vegetables for them. Agnes hypothesized that her own upbringing was central to the development of her relationship with food: "Maybe because the taste is there, maybe because we were raised on a farm."

In Halifax, Nellie Harvey (forty-five, white, lower middle class) also reflected on the influences of her upbringing in discussing her adult preferences. When asked if she ate from a variety of ethnic cuisines, Nellie replied,

> Not for me. I'm pretty well just a basic eater. Try a little bit of spice, not much. My husband's more adventurous than I am, much. He likes sushi and curries and that kind of stuff. I wasn't raised that way, and I don't care for the taste of sushi. I find curry can be a little overpowering. And, you know, it's just what you're accustomed to.

Nellie's family grew apples and pressed them to make their own juice. She recalled, "I remember the first time I tasted processed apple juice, I thought somebody had peed as a joke and that's what they were serving. It just was pathetic. It was horrid. I spit my first mouthful out because it was so foreign from what we had." This aversion signifies deeply embodied tastes. Nellie does not drink apple juice today.

Natalia Warshawski (forty-seven, white, lower middle class) agreed about the tastes learned at home, though she noted that they could change over time: "I think the taste that we grew up with something is really important, yeah. You know, like spiciness. I mean, my parents don't have spice, but I mean we've adapted that now." She reflected on how she and her husband had influenced their children's taste, instilling preferences simply by exposure:

> It's interesting the way they've picked up our habits. I mean, we like Diet Coke; that's the pop that we drink. They don't even look at Pepsi, because that's the beverage that we've always had in the house if we're going to have pop. So they're kind of used to

that, and they're not used to Pepsi. So it's interesting how we've influenced their taste that way.

Teaching taste infuses foods with value-laden meanings. Children learn what "good" food is, where the definition of good is classed, gendered, ethnically marked, and linked to place. As discussed in Chapter 1, most Canadians inextricably link good food to dominant discourses of healthy eating. When asked to define it, they immediately mention healthfulness. Nevertheless, good food is broader, extending beyond nutrition. How food makes us feel, the embodied knowledge of food, can affect how people conceptualize good food, quite apart from notions of health. For many families, the values being embodied along with taste were explicit, especially concerning homemade food and family meals. Notice how sixteen-year-old Nils Wilkinson (white, upper middle class) linked home, family, and social class with taste: "Chicken soup is, like, rainy-day food when you want to warm up. And pot roast is definitely, like, a family, like something that the mom makes, good like a nice home. Yeah. Like a middle-class home and the mom, like, my mom – that's, like, something my mom would make."

Teaching taste is an implicit practice of socialization, as children imbibe ideas along with physical sensations, creating an embodied way of knowing and being. This process is evocatively described by Nadia Seremetakis (1994, 26–30), who depicts a woman feeding her grandchild: through this repetitive everyday practice, the child is nourished and a social identity is created, with sensibilities that are culturally embedded. Among our participants, the conflation of taste with specific values regarding good food frequently drew on the ideal of homemade food and eating at home. For example, Brogan Voisey (thirteen, Irish and Eastern European Canadian, working poor/ impoverished) said, "I like stuff that's not fake. I like stuff that's, like, yummy," such as homemade macaroni and cheese because "it just tastes better and it's like a better – like, it tastes like real cheese."

As noted above, for the Aronowitz family, good food was tasty food procured close to home. Even when she was pushed for time, Agnes prepared homemade meals rather than enjoying the convenience of prepared or processed foods because she considered homemade far superior:

> Oh, we never buy pizza. We always – when all of the kids were
> home a number of years ago, we used to have Friday nights, if
> we were all home, as pizza night. I would make the crust, and we
> would all be in the kitchen, slicing, and everybody would make
> their own crust, and they could throw on whatever they wanted.

She also mentioned making her own version of Hamburger Helper and
cooking burgers and fries herself (rather than going to McDonald's)
on what they called "McAronowitz night." Through everyday food
practices, Agnes was teaching her children particular values – not
only that good food was made at home and that time constraints
did not have to impair quality, but also that certain flavours of fresh-
ness and quality taste good, and *are* good, with an implicit moral
judgment attached.

Nuala Haldane (forty, white, working class) implied that good
foods were homemade but also suggested that good meals were family
meals: "We always ate together at supper. Always. We sat at the kitchen
table, and we all ate together. And my mother always made sure we
had good meals." Nuala saw the family environment as the place
where good food was consumed, reflecting the social value and importance of connecting with others through food.

As a child, Noemi Henderson (forty-two, white, upper middle class)
had learned the value of family meals, a lesson she passed along to her
own children:

> When I grew up, we always sat at the table as a group. Now, I
> come from a divorced family, so it wasn't like the nuclear family
> unit. But it was always with a parent and my siblings. That was
> an important part of the day, is that twenty minutes or whatever
> it would take you to gobble down your food. So it's something I
> wanted to do for my kids.

The teaching of values alongside feeding the family can be quite
explicit. Like Noemi and Nuala, Natalia Warshawski wanted her children to value family meals, but she also wanted to teach them table
manners and to see food in terms of aesthetics (see Chapter 6). She
did this through ambience:

I think food should be an experience. I think it should be more than just meeting the need, more than just a service that's provided. It needs to be time to talk and stuff like that. So yes, I think food is – ambience is important. Actually, we used to eat with candlelight quite a bit ... The kids used to behave better. Yeah, they would, when we had candles it could be macaroni and cheese, and if I turned the lights down, put candles on, it would be a different environment.

Clearly, more abstract lessons may accompany the embodiment of taste. Recall from Chapter 4 that when teens adopted vegetarianism, some parents supported their autonomous decision making, whereas others did not. Thus, lessons about choice and autonomy versus respect for authority may be served along with family meals. Consider Amelia Albert's family, with two teens. Amelia (forty-one, white, lower middle class) described its highly collaborative approach to decision making, as she sought to satisfy everyone's tastes:

If they don't want it, I've said, "Don't lie to me, be honest. Because if you tell me you like it, I will keep making it and putting it in front of you. But if you tell me not so much, you didn't care for that one –." So when I try a new recipe and everybody's eating it, then I say I'll do it again. I think they're being honest with me.

Compare her attitude to that of Kelsey Kidston (forty-two, white, working poor/impoverished), whom we met in Chapter 4. Her response to thirteen-year-old Kaleigh's interest in vegetarianism was, "Well, you're not gonna be a vegetarian."

The chapter on vegetarian eating also reminds us that transmission of taste within families is not seamless. There are definite developmental limitations, as most families described children as "picky eaters" when they were young. Like the vegetarian teens in Chapter 4, children may resist the preferred tastes of their parents and may develop new predilections as they grow. Chapter 6 highlights the ways in which adults may reject and distance themselves from the embodied tastes of their upbringing. As people begin to move in social contexts (Bourdieu 1984) outside the home, they encounter new practices and messages that may (or may not) fit with their primary habitus. Netty Howell (sixty-two, white, working poor/impoverished) described this beautifully. A firm believer in healthy and ethical eating, she carefully passed this commitment on to her children – at first. She found it impossible to sustain after they started school:

> Once the first one went off to school, things changed. The second one didn't eat nearly as purely as the first child did, because the home had already been inundated with, you know, other things had become introduced by the first child. But, you know, I didn't have the control. [He would] come home with ideas about food and say, "I don't really want tofu. I want a hamburger" ... The exposure at school changed everything.

Similarly, Agnes Aronowitz recognized the impact of mass marketing and peer pressure on the children at the school where she taught: "You want to have that because you think it's attractive. Your buddy has that, and your buddy says it's good, and you wanna be like him ... It's the marketing."

CULTIVATING TASTE THROUGH ETHICAL EATING

For some participants, "good eating" was synonymous with ethical eating (see Chapter 2), which was a way of drawing social distinctions linked to class status. Many of these individuals argued that the ethics of food were embodied in the taste. Ardith Elliott (fifty-five, white, working class), for example, bought organic and free-range eggs and chicken, maintaining that they tasted much better than the supermarket equivalents. The yolks of free-range eggs were "a very different colour. They're brighter yellow or orange." She also participated in a farm-share program for organic produce, which she described as "so much better" than non-organic "because it's organic, it's fresh, it's really, really good." Asked if she could tell a difference by taste, she replied, "Oh, yeah, much better."

Ardith's daughter, Ashley (sixteen), echoed her mother's sentiments regarding organic food: "It does taste better and it makes you feel better. It's not half real chicken and half fake chicken." These comments speak to a holistic perception of good eating, where foods embody the soil, sun, and water that individuals can taste, smell, and see as they consume (Trubek 2008). This may be particularly salient for those, such as farming families, who have a strong connection to place, but it was also markedly present in families whose eating practices drew on distinctions of Taste that were grounded in the ethical eating repertoire, which emphasizes organic, local, sustainable, fairly traded, nonprocessed food.

In most families, teens seemed to reiterate their parents' overall approaches to food. Such was the case for twelve-year-old Tawna Parsons, mentioned in Chapter 2, who was highly informed about and supportive of ethical eating. But the teaching and learning of Taste as a form of social distinction was not seamless. Netty Howell, whose case study appeared in Chapter 6, displayed intense commitment to ethical and healthy eating, and insisted that she could taste the difference when foods were produced ethically: "If I put two carrots on the table, and you took a bite and chewed them carefully, both of them, you'd be able to tell without any question which one was the organic carrot." When her eighteen-year-old son, Nolan, was asked if he shared her approach, he replied, "No. I'd like to 'cause, I mean, I know it's the best way to eat. But I don't know, I guess I'm too impulsive or something. I only eat what tastes good all the time." Remarking that his own eating practices concentrated on junk food and fast food, he dismissed ethical eating as a "hard-core organic hippy thing" and avoided it because "it's such a damn trend right now ... A lot of people are doing this 'cause it's really cool. That's annoying."

Yet his later comments seemed to indicate that he may indeed share his mother's values. He said he was far too lazy to walk to the farmers' market or to shops owned by local producers, but he believed that patronizing them was morally superior, as a form of resistance to capitalist economy: "It's a hell of a lot better to buy from Farmer Clem down the road than some guy who's sitting on his fat ass, smoking cigars. Basically, people who already have way more money than they need. So it makes sense to me."

Nolan also mentioned air pollution levels and acid rain in Nova Scotia, noting that he would buy more organic food if he could afford it. He expressed his preference in terms of taste, virtually echoing his mother: "Yeah, no, I like to do that, to buy that stuff. 'Cause it even tastes better. Like, a carrot from the [farmers'] market tastes way better than a carrot from the Superstore."

CULTIVATING TASTE THROUGH COSMOPOLITAN EATING

A common way in which food and tastes are appreciated is through the cuisines and flavours of ethnocultural traditions. After all, combinations of spices, seasonings, and foods create sensory boundaries (albeit porous ones) that serve to categorize ethnicity. As we saw in Chapter 8, for migrants to Canada, maintaining the familiar taste sensations of "home" provides a key means of transmitting cultural membership and belonging across generations. The Esani family (introduced in Chapter 5) had migrated to Canada from Pakistan less than ten years before the interviews, and the children, Aarya, Amara, and Arjan, were quite articulate regarding how tastes not only marked identity, but could be modified to assist performances of belonging, or crossing ethnocultural boundaries. They described Pakistani cuisine as "brown food," defined as "curry, rice, roti, pita," and asserted that "hard-core brown food" could not be adulterated by serving it with "Western" foods such as pasta. Although Pakistani food was central to the performance of their ethnic identities, they emphasized their Western taste preferences when they were feeding friends, fostering ethnocultural boundary crossing and inclusion through demonstrating the breadth of their embodied tastes.

For migrants, "ethnic" grocery stores and restaurants may serve as important spaces to connect with home, in part through their spatial aesthetics (Mankekar 2005). They can establish sensory spaces that evoke the sights (via cultural artifacts and pictures), sounds (music), scents, and tastes of home. They may provide safe space to perform one's ethnocultural Tastes. Yet some study participants found them problematic, as their alterations of taste may compromise perceived authenticity. Adeela Esani (forty-one, South Asian Canadian, upper middle class) said that the sole Pakistani restaurant in her community had begun catering to Western and other South Asian tastes: "He doesn't make food the taste that we would want." Thus, restaurants that represent one's own culinary heritage may provide a taste of the familiar but also the unfamiliar. Here performance of taste and Taste intersect in a particular manner: food may provide a way to perform group membership but also a critique of group construction through a recognition of the myriad, intermingling sensory borders.

Willingness to cross boundaries may indicate one's worldliness or openness to ethnic Others, in a display of cosmopolitanism. Performance of Taste frequently entails an embodied knowledge beyond the final gustatory experiences of consumption, including a physical comprehension and comfort with procurement and preparation. To move comfortably through an ethnic grocery store or restaurant, for example, can evoke the simultaneous comfort and discomfort that accompany navigating ethnic boundaries and unobtrusively observing the rules of interaction.

Since the connoisseur mode of cosmopolitan eating is associated with the upper classes (see Chapter 3), consuming the tastes of the Other can signify elite social status (Heldke 2003). Some participants made a point of this and of cultivating it in their children. Nigel Wood (forty-five, white, upper middle class), for instance, habitually ordered unfamiliar items in restaurants, to experience new tastes: "I go to restaurants in foreign countries and I look at the menu, and if I don't know what it is, I order it. That's how I ate horse in Italy." He found food conservatism narrow and insular, quite distasteful:

> I think it's most important to have an appreciation of food and not be stuck in this "I must eat my cheeseburger exactly the way everyone ever has." It just annoys me. It's like never moving out of your hometown. It's like living in your parents' basement ... Get out and see the world. Do things. And eating's a big part of that.

Not surprisingly, Nigel was extremely proud that his teen daughters would "eat anything," from sushi to dim sum to haggis: "We were eating barbequed chicken feet at the dim sum restaurant, and there's no squeamishness. My younger daughter was probably the only kid in the history of [her] school to bring oxtails and sauerkraut in her lunch."

Many parents who adopted the connoisseur approach inculcated preferences for diverse foods in their children and were proud when they displayed markers of Taste by opting for exotic, authentic flavours rather than mass-produced ones. Belva and Brent Vernon (fifty and fifty-three, white, upper middle class), who were featured in Chapter 3 as exemplifying connoisseur cosmopolitan eating, attempted to cultivate sophisticated palates in their teen sons. Rather than capitulating to youthful "pickiness," as so many parents mentioned, Belva worked hard to teach her sons to like new foods, expanding their preferences:

> I try when I'm planning meals to make sure that everyone's going to love something. So if I know that they both aren't crazy about bulghar, I'll make sure that if we have tabhouli that there's something else that they do like as well. And so, I expect them to taste a bit of everything that's there, but they can fill up on something else … And eventually, they'll love tabhouli too.

She and her husband, Brent, were proud of their teen sons' food adventurousness. They spoke of taking the boys to a French bistro for a celebratory meal and seemed very pleased that their favourite restaurant was Alsatian. Brent pointed to the success of their approach, as indicated by their sons' lack of interest in fast food: "And now they don't want to go to McDonald's. We've never been there. There's never ever, ever, ever a desire to go to McDonald's."

Boyd (sixteen) and Blake (fourteen) agreed with their parents' approach to culinary sophistication:

BOYD: We've always, like, been asked to try, try a bit. Since we were little, I guess, right? Try some, you might like it.
BLAKE: You have to at least try things, yeah.
BOYD: After ten tries –
BLAKE: You'll like –
BOYD: You'll enjoy it or something.

Later Blake reiterated, "We've been brought up to eat everything, or try it."

The importance of cultivating Taste as a form of class distinction was evident in Belva Vernon's comment that Blake was allergic to *cheap* chocolate: "Blake used to be allergic to cheap chocolate. His ears used to go bright red and hot. So we had to fill out those kind of forms you have to send to school where they said, 'Is there an allergy?' and we would just have to put 'cheap chocolate but can tolerate Callebaut' *[laughs]*." Though presented with humour, this anecdote is the ultimate depiction of embodied Taste – only the finest Belgian chocolate will suffice for this fourteen-year-old.

CULTIVATING TASTE THROUGH HEALTHY EATING

For most families, good eating was at least partially linked to conceptions of healthy eating. Yet, as discussed in Chapter 1, healthy eating extends far beyond mere nutrition. Previous chapters have shown that particular discourses of healthy eating can be used to relay messages about social identity, to make distinctions, and to convey judgments about moral superiority and inferiority. Healthy eating, as embodied taste, is one of the markers available for engagement with social hierarchies.

We saw in Chapter 1 that women may constitute themselves as good mothers by instructing their families regarding healthy eating. Not surprisingly, then, the female participants in several of the above examples were attempting to teach their children about good eating in terms of health. We repeatedly heard from teens that they had learned most of what they knew about healthy eating from their mothers and, to a lesser extent, from school. As Blaine Fredericks (fifteen, white, lower middle class) commented about healthy eating, "I probably wouldn't know very much. If I knew anything, it would probably just be from my parents. Maybe a tiny bit from foods class."

Recall from Chapter 1 Bree and Boyd Fagan's intensive approach to eating, in which taste was a distant second to healthiness. As Bree stated, "Taste is just a habit." Their attitude was wholeheartedly supported by their sixteen-year-old daughter, Beata (Swiss Canadian, lower middle class). She did not always make healthy choices, but like her parents she took full responsibility for her decisions and for any negative health consequences. She believed that she and her two siblings had health issues when they ate "bad" foods. She was quite critical of the families of friends who served food that did not meet the Fagans' standards. Discussing a friend who ate too much dairy, Beata said, "Ewww, it's just so unhealthy!" She saw her commitment to healthy eating as a central part of her identity, one that she experienced as fully embodied: "I like eating healthy food because it makes me feel better, plain and simple. I just feel better when I eat well. When I eat junk, I feel it, I know. I want to go sleep."

Whereas for some individuals, healthy eating was synonymous with tasty food, many others constructed healthy food as not tasting particularly good. Taste as gustatory sensation, then, was a basis for resistance – especially by teens – to the Taste of healthy eating, the potential for distinction through moral superiority. For example, Nolan Howell (eighteen, white, working poor/impoverished) loved the taste of unhealthy food, even though it affected his mood: "It gives you a high and then you – I get depressed when I eat McDonald's actually ... I do all kinds of things that I know affect me badly ... But it tastes good. Chips taste great ... Instant gratification." Ashley Elliott (sixteen, white, working class) also found it difficult to resist unhealthy food, simply because it tasted good: "I'm not very healthy. I'd probably be like fifty-fifty because I want to eat healthy, but I also have food cravings and I don't like the food that's healthy most of the time, because I don't find it tastes good." Even Boyd and Blake Vernon, who modelled their cosmopolitan eating on their parents' Tastes, did not always like their mother's healthy cooking. As Blake said, "Well, she prepares healthy, healthy food ... and sometimes her experiments I find aren't very tasty ... And sometimes I wish that there would be a bag of chips just lying there. For when you're, like, needing something like that."

Teaching their children to resist taste preferences in favour of Taste through healthy eating was thus an active pursuit of many mothers. For example, Abby Edward (thirty-six, white, upper middle class) explicitly described shaping her family's preference for the taste of skim milk and whole grains, which she perceived as healthier. Her husband had "converted to the whole wheat side, and he prefers the taste and so do my kids."

Fathers' roles in moulding the palate often seemed to be implicit, modelling behaviour rather than explicitly instilling it, as mothers did. For example, Arlen Evans (eighteen, white, upper middle class) explained that his preferences were the same as his father's: "I have my steaks the same way he does. I have my eggs the same way he does. I like my bacon not really crispy, so kind of on the fatty side, a little bit of chewy side. So I do eat a lot like my dad does, I guess." The process here appears to be teaching by modelling and learning through observation. Nonetheless, Arlen seems to have embraced stereotypical masculine/unhealthy eating (see Chapters 1 and 5), enjoying the taste of "manly" foods – steak and eggs, fatty bacon.

There is no question that substantial lessons about gender roles and expectations are served up with family meals, especially in the inculcation of healthy eating. The typical emphases of healthy eating (light foods, restraint, and portion control) appeared to centre less on taste (as gustatory sensation) and more on Taste (aesthetic, culturally constructed perceptions reflecting particular social norms and values) (Korsmeyer 1999). Healthy food was seen as "good" in ways beyond gustatory enjoyment, relating to other embodied pleasures, particularly that of having a slim, strong, healthy body. In fact, mothers often seemed to be modelling for children – especially daughters – the need to disregard their own desires and tastes in favour of Taste, as a kind of feminine refinement. Although they did most of the foodwork, women frequently ignored their own preferences as a self-disciplinary technique through which they might produce an appropriate (slender) feminine body (see Chapter 5).

Self-denial as an attribute of Taste was highly gendered, in that it was discussed far more by women and girls as a means to attain or maintain slenderness. But as we saw in Chapter 5, some men and boys were also engaged in self-surveillance, a typically feminine preoccupation made more readily available to them through the language of healthy eating and fighting obesity. Blanche Fitzgerald (forty-six, white, upper middle class) was quite concerned about the weight of two of her sons, but she and her husband intentionally framed their concerns around health, rather than weight or body image:

> With the kids, we try not to say things about weight in front of them. We talk about wanting to eat, you know, in a more healthy way. We always phrase it that way when we talk about it. You know, we talk a bit about it I suppose here and there, but we're quite – like, they seem to have pretty healthy ideas about food so far.

Yet Blanche's attempts to instruct her son Brant about healthy eating (to achieve a particular body) were highly intentional. She described a recent meal with him:

> Brant has to be a bit more mindful, I think, because he could easily just blow up because he loves food, so he tends to overeat. He said today when he ate his burger ... 'I hate that I eat so fast.' Because he's starting to notice that his stomach won't feel good at

the end of it because he's eaten really quickly. So I would say to him, 'Well, I've noticed that if you put your fork down in between your bites' – so he was trying that with his pie because, of course, then he still goes on to pie.

This way of eating – setting the fork down between bites – is a clear example of cultivating Taste through conquering desire. Discipline and denial of taste are learned markers of Taste, the distinction that accrues through successful engagement with healthy eating. The intent is that it will eventually be imprinted on the body, through slenderness, which is seen as synonymous with health.

Many participants spoke of the need to resist, avoid, or manage cravings, especially for fatty, salty, and sugary items. Nan Howe (forty-eight, white, working class), for example, managed her cravings for potato chips by eating low-fat baked chips, sacrificing taste for healthfulness: "They aren't as tasty, but I think I'm doing better for myself." Anezka Embler (sixteen, white, upper middle class) noted that stress affected her ability to resist treats: "If I'm especially stressed, I might think I deserve it, but that usually leads to more stress on my part, because I think, 'Oh, now I've blown it.'" Chocolate, chips, cookies, and ice cream were most commonly identified as the objects of craving, thus demanding self-control. There seems to be a reflection here of the social idea that pleasurable sensations are dangerous and must therefore be avoided.

Much has been written on the conflation of sin and morality with the pleasures/dangers of eating, particularly eating certain foods (such as chocolate) (see Coveney 2000; Griffith 2004; Moore 2008). Interestingly, food as gratification and as a tool for coping with stress and depression was articulated by participants of European descent, which may speak to family and cultural histories concerning the moralities of food. In contrast, interviewees who had recently migrated to Canada from non-European locales did not seem to speak of food in this way, perhaps due to their different religious traditions and cultural ways of relating to food. These hints about the ethnocultural moralities of food, however, suggest one way in which taste and Taste intertwine; the taste of food is interpreted as healthy or unhealthy, good or bad, based on Tastes – cultural histories, learned community/

family social values, and individual experiences. In other words, the interpretation of gustatory sensations is grounded in socio-culturally moderated aesthetics and values.

The deliberate inculcating of Taste in terms of healthy eating – teaching youth to curtail food preferences for longer-term status that will be evident on the body – was particularly apparent when parents disagreed regarding food practices. These conflicts were most obvious among divorced parents; typically, mothers complained about ex-husbands who served the children unhealthy food, undermining the project of constructing them as healthy eaters (revealed through slender bodies). For example, Anicka Embler (forty-three, Czech Canadian, upper middle class) recalled her anger when her ex-husband took their young daughter Anezka to McDonald's for adult-sized meals, contributing to her weight gain:

> I was just so frustrated at that time and – her dad. I just tried my best, and she was quite young. I switched her to skim milk. I tried to start teaching her, "You have to take control of how much you eat." Just trying different tactics and stuff. It was just such a frustrating time for me, because it just felt like a losing battle. That was just a very difficult period of time.

Anicka's attempts to teach her daughter Taste, in the sense of light foods, portion control, and the achievement of slenderness, were thwarted by her ex-husband's focus on gustatory taste.

For her part, Anezka (sixteen) saw herself as overweight, which she attributed to her father's influence and his emphasis on pleasure through taste:

> My father was a main influence in that. He was a very unhealthy eater. So whenever I went over to his house, it would be just kind of be the junk food weekend. So my mom tried to mend that, but there's not a whole lot you can do when you're away from the house, so that kind of influenced bad eating from the beginning.

Anezka identified her father's tastes and preference for junk food as characteristic of his own family. She spoke at length about the

Tastelessness of these foods, linking it directly to health and body size, and explicitly describing sensory preferences as learned:

> They're all fairly overweight on that side and greatly enjoy their greasy foods. I think that might be where my father picked that up. So it's kind of a cycle. Just about any unhealthy food you can think of, they'll eat. And their recipes consist of "add butter, add the meat, add more butter, and a whole bunch of salt." And he insists it's part of their heritage, or something weird like that ... From my grandparents to my dad to me – it just kind of has been passed along. And they just kind of view it as the norm.

Anezka described the embodiment of tastes across generations (habitus). At the time of our interviews, she had ended contact with her father, citing food as a critical factor in the conflict: "Food was indeed a big issue there, and he didn't understand that, even in the end." Living full-time with her mother, Anezka was dieting for weight loss, conforming more closely to her mother's food practices and Tastes, which were grounded in the mainstream healthy eating discourse. As she altered her diet, she was breaking bonds with her father's foodways and cultivating a new palate.

Like Anicka Embler, Ardith Elliott (fifty-five, white, working class) was frustrated by her ex-husband's insistence on privileging taste over health and quality, which she saw as having embodied consequences for their children: "[He] would take them out and give them pop and stuff that I wasn't allowing them to have at all. And that was a problem for me, because I did see behaviour issues with them, and I was the one who got handed them back at the end of the night, after they'd had sugar and deep-fried stuff."

Ardith's daughter Ashley (sixteen) had internalized her perceptions of good food. Although she liked the taste of the energy-dense, high-fat, processed and fast foods that her father preferred, they left her feeling "tired and stuff." In contrast, when she followed her mother's healthy eating Tastes, "The more fresh I eat, the better I feel." She concluded, "I wouldn't want to eat completely at my dad's house, because I would eventually feel fat, like, health-wise."

As Ashley struggled with the tension between Taste and taste, trying to respect the symbolic and moral boundaries of good eating, she felt considerable guilt for desiring foods that her mother deemed bad, even Tasteless:

> I like having treats ... My mom doesn't buy things other than popsicles ... I like a little bit of ketchup chips. I'm really into soft drinks and Slurpees. I try to get the small ones. I get the small bags of ketchup chips. I don't get the big one. I like it. I think that's the only kind of chips I really like. And they're not even very good. It's, like, I just eat them because I want them.

Ashley felt unable to ask her mother to purchase "bad" foods, such as chips, even if she herself paid for them, so she sometimes walked to the corner store and bought them on the sly, nervously enjoying the flavours in the privacy of her own room. Note that even as she savoured her guilty pleasures, Ashley employed the technique of self-discipline, through portion control. She was learning to embody Taste, as taught through the discourse of healthy eating.

Bodily sensations are physically experienced, but how they are interpreted, perceived, and understood is culturally constructed. The sense of both taste and Taste (Korsmeyer 1999) are taught. The palate is moulded, a result of physical sensations and experiences with socio-cultural aesthetics that are implicitly and explicitly taught. Family is the primary locus where this process occurs, which explains why the tastes of childhood are so poignant.

CONCLUSION

More than any other in the book, this chapter highlights the body. Yet the body is not separate from the socio-cultural relationships to food that were discussed in previous chapters. Rather, it is the means through which social and cultural influences operate. The intersections of class, place, gender, and food practices are embodied experiences.

This chapter explored how the habitus (Bourdieu 1984) is learned and taught, noting that particular understandings of and relationships to food enter bodies, even as everyday eating practices become embedded in sensory selves. The teaching of taste, the inculcation of the habitus, is primarily informal and unintended. Gustatory taste, and with it particular notions of what constitutes good food and good eating, is learned implicitly in the family home, through physical sensations. It becomes embodied.

The inculcation of Taste, the culturally constructed perceptions of food and eating practices (Korsmeyer 1999), is often more deliberate. Through it, we learn to perform particular relationships to food that indicate our social position. Notions of good eating incorporate performances of self that convey place, class, and gender, through distinctions of Taste (Bourdieu 1984). The evaluations of self and Others that are enabled through the discourses of healthy, ethical, and cosmopolitan eating make available particular cultural repertoires for instructing young people on Taste. Not surprisingly, friction may arise when parents' tastes and Tastes differ. These tensions may become embodied in children, who struggle with conflicting teachings, emotions, and connections through food.

Place also plays a role in embodied performances of taste/Taste. For migrants, gustatory sensations can evoke yearning for the taste of home, which may co-exist in complex tension with the desire for the tastes of "here," the new place, which has its own rules of engagement for food. For some, tasting the exotic, authentic Other embodies the performance of cosmopolitanism and elite social status. Some parents quite deliberately cultivated this Taste in their children.

The relationship between good, tasty eating, and discourses of healthy eating is equally complex. For some, healthy food simply tasted better. For others, the enjoyment of "forbidden" items overrode intellectual knowledge about what is "good for" us, and healthy foods were equated with lack of taste. Gustatory pleasure thus became grounds for resistance to healthy eating discourses.

Resistance to healthy eating simultaneously resists the self-discipline demanded of "good" eaters. It is both highly gendered and connected to life stage. Teen boys learn to embody masculinity by cultivating a taste for "unhealthy eating" (the habitus). Teen girls learn to embody a culturally specific and classed femininity by opting for light, healthy eating. Their performance of Taste is centred in part on denying their own desires. As Charlotte Biltekoff (2013) and Deborah McPhail (2009) suggest in their critical examinations of healthy eating and anti-obesity discourses, conquering the foibles of the weak-willed body, mastering discipline and self-control, can be constructed not only as markers of class and masculinity, but also as patriotism in national projects to strengthen the populace in the face of vague external threats. Conquering the body (gustatory taste) in favour of Taste signifies success – at individual, collective, and even national scales.

conclusion

THIS BOOK OPENED with a series of questions: How did you and your household decide what to eat today? How do your finances and the availability of food determine your daily approach to meals? Do ideas about "normal" eating, class, ethnicity, and gender play a role in your decisions? How do you use food to convey your social identity? How do you use it to mark symbolic boundaries – or make moral judgments – about others whose eating habits differ from yours?

The goal of the research presented in this book was to make sense of the everyday eating practices of Canadians from varied social and geographic locations, focusing on the intersections of class, place, and gender in family food practices. Using social science theoretical frameworks and qualitative research methods, we interviewed people in four regions of Canada. We talked to them about what they did and did not eat, and what they thought about their own eating habits and those of others. We analyzed what they said (and did not say) to uncover the cultural logics that underpin food practices. Our aim was to explore how the conscious, semi-conscious, and unconscious influences that shape what people say and do in relation to food are grounded in the social contexts of their lives and bound up in their social identities.

The preceding chapters explored specific themes that emerged from the research, beginning with healthy eating. All participants were familiar with this, and it figured prominently in their evaluation of their own eating practices and those of others. Differing definitions of healthy eating appeared to be related to where interviewees lived and to their class and economic context, but gender was clearly the dominant social category here. Concerns about ethical eating were less ubiquitous than those about healthy eating but were also shaped by class and geographic context. An interest in cosmopolitan eating was not exclusive to socio-economic elites but was linked to the economic and cultural resources that a family commanded. Subsequent chapters examined the way in which healthy, ethical, and cosmopolitan eating played out in connection with vegetarianism, body image, changing social and geographic contexts, and through embodied eating experiences.

THE CULTURAL LOGICS OF FOOD PRACTICES

The chapters in this book have documented the varied ways in which food practices are shaped by social location and used to construct identities. The cultural and symbolic capital (Bourdieu 1984) associated with certain ways of eating allows people to draw boundaries through food choices, distinguishing themselves from social others (Lamont 2000). At the same time, performances of identities are not completely scripted and pre-determined by factors such as class or gender. The multiple cultural repertoires that are available to people allow for tremendous variety in the ways they eat and the food issues they discuss, despite the pervasive influence of social locations (Swidler 1986).

Gender and Food Practices

Gender had arguably the greatest influence on participant engagement with food, despite some reluctance to acknowledge or discuss its impact. Our data strongly suggest that feeding families is still primarily women's domain. In recruiting study participants, we asked to interview as many eligible family members as possible; despite our best efforts, we usually ended up interviewing an adult woman and one or more teen children. In only 18 of our 105 families (at least 65 of which included an adult male) did an adult man agree to be interviewed. In all these families, his female partner also participated. Typically, he was not comfortable with being interviewed alone, and so was interviewed jointly with his partner. We also noted that in almost all families, an adult woman was primarily responsible for planning menus, shopping for groceries, cooking, and orchestrating meals that balanced individual preferences, busy schedules, and cultural traditions. In this regard, the gendered nature of family food-work seems to have changed very little during the past several decades (DeVault 1991; Lupton 2001). Our data also revealed that women's responsibilities extended beyond ensuring that everyone was fed to caring for everyone's health (see Beagan et al. 2008; Biltekoff 2013). This was intimately bound up in their presentation of self as moral citizens (Foucault 1991) and their marking of the symbolic boundaries between their social identities and those of others (Lamont 2000). By promoting the principles of healthy eating and incorporating healthy foods into family meals, women could establish an identity that was recognizably feminine, mark themselves as good mothers, and distinguish themselves from women whom they critiqued as inadequately feeding themselves and their families.

The intertwining of performance of gender with engagement in healthy eating also involved body weight and appearance management. Healthy eating was equated with light eating, weight loss, and control of fat and calorie intake – traditionally associated with the enactment of femininity. Although widely circulated feminist analyses (see Chernin 1985; Wolf 1992; Bordo 1993; Rice 2007) have provided women with a critical perspective on physical ideals and dieting, these have been challenged during the past decade by even more widely disseminated rhetoric regarding rising obesity rates and associated health problems. Thus, though women and teenage girls may avoid the language of "dieting," that of "healthy eating" can signify similar preoccupations with self-governance and appearance, reproducing traditional patterns of femininity. These concerns are not value-neutral, as shown by female interviewees who conveyed a sense of guilt when they "confessed" to eating junk foods and who described healthy eating in terms of virtuousness.

In contrast, men's performances of masculinity were perhaps best demonstrated through their non-participation in the research, as mentioned above. A closer look at their involvement and non-involvement shows that associations between masculinity and food are moderated by social class. Although our interviewees came from a range of classes, all but one of the eighteen men were either upper (twelve) or lower (five) middle class.* Their higher cultural and economic capital was associated with greater freedom in their enactment of masculinity, allowing them to express an interest in food that deviated from hegemonic masculinity's focus on meat, hearty meals, and general indifference to cooking (other than barbequing!) (Mróz et al. 2011b). Some men were highly engaged with connoisseur cosmopolitanism. Their focus on aesthetic appreciation of food, showcasing expert knowledge and seeking exotic, authentic dishes, was grounded in an alternative masculinity that has been noted elsewhere as signifying class-based distinctions and distance from necessity (Bourdieu 1984; Wandel and Roos 2005). Even these men, however, demonstrated little involvement with (and sometimes active resistance to) healthy eating, indicating the strength of its association with femininity. However, societal concerns linking increasing obesity rates to chronic disease seem to be weakening this resistance somewhat, initiating more men and boys into weight control by allowing them to frame it in relation to health rather than appearance (Monaghan 2008; Norman 2013).

Interestingly, despite the prominence of gender in shaping participants' engagement with food and their ability to identify stereotypical feminine and masculine ways of eating, they were reluctant to associate their own food practices with gender. Instead, they ascribed what might be seen as gendered practices to individual preference. We argue that this denial of gender and individualizing of tastes strengthens inequities by allowing gender disparities to go "underground," making it difficult to organize for systemic change (Beagan et al. 2008; McPhail, Beagan, and Chapman 2012).

Social Class and Food Practices

Throughout the study, we saw numerous instances of food practices as markers of symbolic boundaries, drawing both moral and cultural

. . . .

* The remaining man, a working-class member of a conservative cultural group, attended the first interview only, apparently to vet the involvement of his wife and daughter.

distinctions (Lamont 2000). Participants from lower classes tended to make a virtue of necessity, placing a high value on frugality and eating plain, simple, hearty, filling food. In contrast, those from higher classes were more likely to employ cultural boundaries that valorized pleasure, aesthetics, adventure, expert knowledge, and the consumption of ethical foods.

These divisions were clear in our analyses of ethical and cosmopolitan eating, which our middle-class interviewees employed to assert distinction and cultural capital. It was primarily the middle-class – and mostly upper-middle-class – participants who were strongly engaged with dominant ethical eating practices such as environmental sustainability and supporting local farmers. Similarly, they were most highly engaged in connoisseur cosmopolitan eating, seeking out new, exotic foods, esoteric culinary knowledge, and authentic food experiences. Middle-class families seemed most readily able to access the cultural repertoires of mainstream ethical eating and connoisseur cosmopolitanism.

In contrast, participants from less privileged social positions, closer to necessity, were more likely to creatively adapt dominant ethical eating practices to fit their incomes and to engage with alternative ethical and moral frameworks, such as recycling and reducing waste, food security, or caring for the food and social needs of others in their community. When they did undertake cosmopolitan eating, their approach was pragmatic and more tentative. Pragmatic cosmopolitans interacted with diverse cuisines through their exposure in diverse urban neighbourhoods and social circles; they were often open to new culinary experiences, but they did not usually seek out education or expertise concerning exotic cuisines. Tentative cosmopolitans were ambivalent about new cuisines and dishes, desiring to stay connected with familiar tastes or foods of their youth. Though not objectively superior, the practices of the upper classes tend to be granted greater cultural and symbolic capital.

Such was the case with vegetarianism. Parents who supported teen vegetarianism were currently or had previously been in middle- and upper-middle class locations. This links to the above discussion of ethical and connoisseur cosmopolitan eating as markers of middle-class habitus – vegetarianism maps onto ethical concerns about environmental sustainability and animal welfare, as well as the connoisseur cosmopolitan practice of seeking out new dishes, food-related information, and cooking techniques. It can also map onto mainstream and alternative understandings of healthy eating (lower fat, emphasis on plant-based dishes). It might also be seen as requiring that considerable time and attention be devoted to food, typically a more elite culinary practice. Only working-class and low-income families resisted teen vegetarianism, opting instead for the traditional view that a healthy diet included meat. Parents who opposed teen vegetarianism often enacted particular approaches to raising children, in which protecting their nutritional health trumped encouraging their autonomous decision making.

Participants who had moved from one class location to another also used food and eating practices to communicate classed identities. In many instances, they drew boundaries that made a virtue of their own practices and moral stances – whether these originated from their former or current class location – distinguishing themselves from Others with different class histories. Regardless of their class trajectory, virtually all these interviewees employed the healthy eating discourse to castigate the food practices of Others – the "unhealthy" lower classes they had left behind or whose ranks they had joined due to downward mobility. Either way, healthy eating was a means of distinguishing from the class of origin or current class location.

For those with limited access to cultural and economic capital, evoking frugality seemed to be the only other way of exhibiting moral worth. In contrast, those who were further from necessity could employ the various aspects of ethical and cosmopolitan eating to display their membership in higher classes and to distance themselves from the lower ones. When a participant's class position changed, the food practices of childhood no longer suited the new social and economic circumstances. Some individuals – especially those with an upward trajectory – easily adopted the practices of their new class. Others, however, could not abandon the habits of childhood. Among these were upwardly mobile people whose frugality impeded the purchase of expensive organic, fair-trade food, and those with a downward trajectory who persisted in buying ethical food despite not being able to afford it. At times, these participants recognized the resultant tension, either as an internal unease or as a discomfort that played out in family relationships. Notably, participants retained the class-based dispositions to which they attached moral virtue, not the ones they saw as inferior.

Place and Food Practices

The link between eating practices and geographic location was an important focus of this study. Thus, to explore how eating was characteristic of locale, we recruited families that were clustered in certain areas. The ten study sites were chosen to include four distinct regions of Canada and from rural communities, towns, small to mid-sized cities, and large metropolitan centres.

Not surprisingly, we found considerable evidence of interrelationships among the foods available in an area, the food repertoires in residents' cultural tool kits, and the eating practices that people described as typical of the community. Availability of ethical foods facilitated higher engagement with the dominant discourse of ethical eating. Interviewees saw this version of ethical eating as very well supported in certain areas: they particularly referred to Vancouver but also mentioned Kingston and some parts of Toronto as having ready availability of local, organic, and fair-trade products as well as the social interactions that support ethical eating. Similarly, abundance of "authentic" foods from a multitude of ethnic cuisines, personal connections to people from varied cultural backgrounds, and social circles where new and exotic dishes were regularly shared were all commonly associated with connoisseur cosmopolitan eating. Living in neighbourhoods where other people were seen to be involved in and supportive of ethical or cosmopolitan eating encouraged engagement with these repertoires (see also Johnston, Rodney, and Szabo 2012).

Through these kinds of interactions, geographic location was able to moderate some of the class-specific logics discussed above. For example, though connoisseur cosmopolitan eating was usually seen in middle-class families, lower-income interviewees who lived in Toronto and Vancouver (and to a lesser extent, Edmonton) could easily engage in a pragmatic cosmopolitanism that relied on personal connections with people from varied backgrounds. In contrast, lower-income participants who lived in rural areas did not have the same exposure to diverse people and foods, and thus did not demonstrate the pragmatic cosmopolitanism of urban centres. The moderating effect of place also applied when access to economic and cultural capital mitigated the limitations of geographic amenities. Well-off interviewees compensated for rural lack of diversity through travel and gastronomic leisure pursuits. In a reverse scenario, lack of income might impede the ability to take advantage of the healthy ways of eating that characterized a neighbourhood.

Although participants made fewer distinctions between regions than we had originally expected, rural-urban differences were striking (and within them, gradations between towns, cities, and metropolitan centres). Rural areas were sometimes idealized, and urban-dwellers who had migrated to the country appreciated the increased availability, quality, and authenticity of homegrown, homemade food, as well as knowing the local producers. However, many interviewees commented that long-term locals did not appreciate these things, mostly eating processed food from supermarkets. Participants who lived in urban centres, or had done so, generally denigrated rural culinary repertoires as dull, outdated, unhealthy, unsophisticated, and resistant to change. Rural people were characterized as not caring about healthy eating, despite their ready access to fresh, local, natural, homegrown items. In contrast, urban culinary repertoires and eating practices (except for those of Halifax) were generally portrayed as healthy, cosmopolitan, multicultural, varied, and superior to those of the country.

These urban-rural distinctions almost perfectly mirrored the class distinctions described earlier. Urban physical and social environments were seen as places where people enacted repertoires of connoisseur cosmopolitanism, dominant modes of ethical eating, and conspicuous healthy eating. All of these typify middle- and upper-middle-class dispositions, so they convey greater cultural capital than repertoires associated with working- and lower-class dispositions. The association of urban spaces with the preferences and embodied practices of higher classes affords these spaces greater cultural capital. Interactions between geography and social class can thus be interpreted in relation to Bourdieu's (1986) conceptualization regarding the interaction of types of capital. The working-class and working-poor families of urban and rural areas may be alike in their low economic capital, but the former could enjoy the greater cultural capital that is associated with the food practices of cities. Well-off rural residents could use their economic capital to "buy" the cultural capital typical of urban food practices.

The higher cultural capital of urban centres also carries symbolic power. Just as food practices mark class distinctions, they also mark hierarchical boundaries between urban and rural. Participants who lived in larger cities, or had done so, particularly used urban-rural distinctions to distance themselves from rural Others, establishing their cultural and moral superiority over long-term rural locals. The rural Others were cast as not appreciating the pastoral context in which they lived, limiting themselves to a bland diet and processed foods. Interestingly, though interviewees in constrained economic circumstances drew moral boundaries to imbue their culinary habits with virtue, those who had always lived in rural communities rarely valorized their own eating practices while belittling those of urbanites. On the whole, they did not make such comparisons.

About Ethnicity

Although our research design did not foreground the interrelationships between food practices and ethnicity, some participants had a wide variety of ethnicities and migration histories. Inevitably, class, gender, ethnicity, and cultural logics of food practices intersect.

The dominant discourses of healthy, ethical, and cosmopolitan eating are undoubtedly linked to ways of performing Euro-Canadian whiteness. All three were arguably less prominent for participants who self-identified as members of minority ethnic groups. Although all interviewees were familiar with notions of healthy eating, ethnic minority participants did not stand out in those conversations. Mothers' concerns about supporting family health and well-being were certainly present. In some families, such as the Esanis in Chapter 5, promoting healthy eating for weight management was an obvious focus and source of tension. But as illustrated in previous research (Ristovski-Slijepcevic, Chapman, and Beagan 2008, 2010; Chapman, Ristovski-Slijepcevic, and Beagan 2011), ethnic minority group members (and recent immigrants in particular) may understand healthy eating in terms of traditional knowledge that is passed down for generations, with some additions (and perhaps contradictions) to the healthy eating discourse that dominates in Canada. Arising as it does from Western science, the mainstream discourse excludes certain aspects of eating that many people see as influencing health (see Biltekoff 2013).

Similarly, the dominant ethical eating repertoire was not particularly reflective of minority views. Almost all participants who were highly involved with this repertoire were Euro-Canadian, whereas racialized migrant families tended to have low to moderate engagement. Interviewees from ethnic minority groups appeared to have less access to the repertoire, opting instead for alternative approaches, which followed different underlying moral frameworks, sometimes based in cultural or religious beliefs. Their version of ethical eating deviated from its dominant counterpart, whose framing of ethics is limited in many ways.

In analyzing cosmopolitan eating, we excluded participants from non-Euro-Canadian backgrounds so we could assess cultural omnivorousness in a homogeneous sample, where the traditional foods of minority ethnic groups can be experienced as exotic, adventurous, and novel. Clearly, such foods often constitute ways of performing ethnic identity for migrants to Canada, through preparing and consuming a "taste of home." At the same time, however, transnational identities (connections to both culture of origin and Western culture) may give rise to particular logics of practice concerning food, as needs and desires around ethnicity and identity performance diverge along lines of age, gender, and class. Adult immigrants in particular may go to great lengths to obtain the flavours of home – increasingly over time, an imagined home – and may hold on to other aspects of ethnic identity embedded in food practices. Their teenaged children, however, may choose to embrace "Canadian" foodways, a dynamic that shapes the complex mix of practices in the performance of transnational identities. Mothers typically assumed primary responsibility for dealing with intergenerational conflicts concerning food, frequently absorbing extra work as they prepared dishes from two or more cultural cuisines to satisfy everyone.

Food Practices in the Family

Finally, our research concentrated on the significance of family contexts and the interpersonal relations experienced there. How are people's everyday food practices developed, negotiated, and resisted in family settings?

Our data provided ample evidence that the family is the primary site where food tastes and dispositions are learned and taught. Although teen participants tended to be less articulate than their mothers regarding what, why, and how they ate, their comments tended to reflect those of their parents. Teen food practices were complex. Participants acknowledged the stereotype of teen consumption as focused on junk food, taste, convenience, and lack of concern for healthy eating, but most of our teen interviewees did not fit this stereotype. Many characterized their own eating habits as mostly healthy, and they appreciated the healthy food and health guidance provided in their homes (see also McPhail, Chapman, and Beagan 2011). Those whose parents prized eclectic tastes and adventurous eating and/or local, organic, and other ethical foods often echoed their values, whereas others appreciated the "normal" meat-and-potatoes cuisine served in their homes.

Some parents (usually mothers) made a concerted effort to inculcate certain Tastes in their children, but much of the teaching and learning appeared to be informal and unconscious, as children observed what and how other family members ate and listened to what their parents said about food. Through this process, they learned to identity "good" food and began to embody the habitus of their parents. At the same time, they embodied broader cultural and familial messages, including values such as the superiority of homemade food, the importance of family meals, the appropriateness of certain behaviours while dining, and convictions about particular approaches to parenting.

Intrafamilial transmission of food practices also encompasses the performance of social identities, displays of social capital, and conveying hierarchical social positions through marking of symbolic boundaries. This form of instruction is sometimes implicit but can be extraordinarily explicit and deliberate. Parents invest in the cultural capital embodied in their children (Cairns, Johnston, and MacKendrick 2013), striving to produce young adults whose class and moral superiority are imprinted on their bodies and indelibly instilled in their palates.

Like their parents, teens used food to distinguish self from Other, conveying their own social position by casting moral judgments on Others (often other teens) whom they characterized as having unhealthy eating habits (see McPhail, Chapman, and Beagan 2011), or not caring about ethical food issues, or as having limited palates. Although gender differences in food practices were not as marked between teen boys and girls as they were between their parents, girls did display some concerns associated with femininity, particularly in relation to body image and the desire to eat low-calorie foods as part of appearance management. Some teens overtly rejected the food-related commitments of their parents, such as dominant versions of ethical eating, yet revealed an underlying belief in them, even as they resisted the attendant everyday practices.

Teaching and learning about taste and Taste often occurred seamlessly, but teens who shuttled between two households sometimes struggled with conflicting emotions and expectations regarding food. Friction also arose in households where teens adopted food preferences and values that differed from those of their parents. This was most visible in some migrant families whose teens resisted daily consumption of ethnic food. Mothers tended to respond by serving some non-traditional dishes, demonstrating that the transmission of food practices in families is negotiated and reciprocal. This also occurred among families who followed a teen's example and adopted a vegetarian diet or reduced their meat consumption. In some families, however, parents resisted teen vegetarianism, especially when it conflicted with their child-rearing style, taste preferences, and familiarity with recipes and cooking techniques, with the result that the teen often returned to meat eating.

Overall, it is clear that feeding a family is not just about providing nutrition or spaces where children can experience social connection, or about creating the social structures that form the family. It is also about transmission of embodied tastes, dispositions, and logics of practice through which people perform their identities and distinguish themselves from others in social hierarchies.

IMPLICATIONS FOR RESEARCH AND THEORY

In her brilliant analysis of four historical food movements, all aimed at encouraging Americans to "eat right," Charlotte Biltekoff (2013) emphasizes that social and cultural mechanisms ensure that ideal diets and body shapes align (seemingly naturally) with the food practices and preferences of the elite. She warns that all members of a society should question common sense assumptions about the moral worth of "good eaters" and beware the condemnation meted out, however unintentionally, to supposedly bad eaters. Her work reveals that dietary discourses such as healthy eating and anti-obesity – but also domestic science in the 1890s, nutritional science during the Second World War, and the alternative food movement of the 1960s and 1970s – can be used in the service of particular race, class, and gender politics, through the construction of the unhealthy Other. She calls on researchers to examine how such dietary reform discourses are taken up by ordinary people. This is precisely what our study has done.

Our work has important implications for research on food practices and consumption more broadly. Methodologically, it illustrates the power of photo-elicitation techniques. Increasingly, researchers are asking participants to capture the difficult-to-articulate by taking photos or at least providing visual cues for more in-depth interviewing. In this study, we wanted to "get at" aspects of food practices that connect to the habitus, to ways of being that are unquestioned and semi-conscious. Taking photos allowed people to show us things that they were not able to talk about, privileging visual over verbal (Power 2003).

What proved even more useful, however, was the less common technique of having participants respond to photos that we showed them. Their own shots remained within their spheres of comfort and familiarity, whereas our photographs moved into areas of potential discomfort and unfamiliarity. They allowed us to reach a gut-level sense of belonging or not belonging in certain food environments, a sense of ease or dis-ease attached to various foods that revealed aspects of habitus and cultural repertoires. Bourdieu (1984, 197) employed the telling comment "That's not for the likes of us" to articulate the way in which tastes and preferences learned in a specific socio-cultural context become internalized, embodied in the habitus, and shared with others in the same social location. Discussing participants' discomfort with a formal French dining room or an inexpensive diner, their aversion to Kraft Dinner or a tiny portion of broiled fish drizzled with a fig balsamic reduction, provided invaluable insight into the operation of habitus in shaping food practices.

Our methods and study design were not without their limitations, and we would do certain things differently in the future. Despite the use of two photo-elicitation techniques, our data consisted primarily of conversations in an interview setting. Both interviews and photo-elicitation involve aspects of performance that may or may not match a person's everyday behaviour (Brown 2009; but see also Pugh 2011). Cultural repertoires, symbolic and moral boundary marking, and performing distinction are all interactional in nature. In interviews, the interaction is primarily with the interviewer, and people undoubtedly performed certain subjectivities for our benefit. Unable to observe participants for an extended period, we inevitably wonder about gaps between their stated and actual practices. To some extent, this limitation was countered by having multiple family members involved in interviews, potentially performing differing scripts. Nonetheless, observational and longitudinal research on family food practices would be invaluable.

Some scholars have questioned the applicability of Bourdieu's (1984) research in 1960s France to other (ostensibly less hierarchically organized) countries more than half a century later (see Bennett et al. 2009; Silva and Warde 2010). Nonetheless, the extent to which his ideas held true in our study was rather remarkable. Whereas the tastes and practices of our elite participants differed from those depicted by Bourdieu, they were still distinct, enjoying a high degree of social legitimacy and providing a significant means to distinguish class. The cultural repertoires of healthy, ethical, and cosmopolitan eating were far more difficult to access for families who lived in poverty.

There is no question that concepts of habitus and disposition, drawn from Bourdieu, help us to make sense of the ways that parents teach and children learn social distinctions, through the development of sensory tastes that come to embody the aesthetics and moral judgments of Taste. The resilience of at least some aspects of the food habitus is evident among those who traverse class boundaries. Yet change inevitably occurs, especially as social fields continually expand and overlap, not least through technologies of travel and communication. Ann Swidler's (1986) insistence on the individual's active agency when engaging with culture, through cultural repertoires, points to how change can arise. Faced with new social circumstances, people dust off little-used elements of their repertoires, using them to navigate the new situation. Adults from farming backgrounds who move to the city may draw on their prior relationship to the land and the act of growing food to successfully navigate dominant discourses of ethical eating, marking themselves as urbane and morally good. Adults who move from working-class to middle-class circumstances, through education, marriage, or both, may draw on their experiences as servers in high-end restaurants to cultivate a level of comfort with elite food practices. Migrants to Canada may employ their familiarity with pizza, an elite dish in their country of origin, to mark their belonging in Western food environs by re-creating it as common fare.

But Foucault's (1979, 1988) notion of discourse also enriches both Bourdieu's concept of embodied dispositions and Swidler's ideas about active engagement with culture. Clearly, dominant discourses such as healthy, ethical, and cosmopolitan eating are used to govern ourselves and others, through surveillance, inspection, examination, and confession. People use food-related discourses as social tools to constitute themselves as "good mothers" or "proper Canadians." They also use dominant discourses to construct their children as infused not only with moral worth, but also with cultural and symbolic capital. The intentionality displayed by parents who sought to cultivate a sophisticated palate or a properly slender "healthy" body in their children indicates not only the power of these discursive constructions, and their connection to symbolic capital, but also the importance of instilling them in the body itself. The body becomes a canvas upon which individuals seek to paint a distillation of discursive power relations, filtered always through available material resources.

The study data provide a valuable example of discourses in action. Although a particular discourse may be dominant at any given time and place, others are always in play, as emergent or alternative discourses. They may or may not eventually garner institutional support to acquire dominance. The mainstream healthy eating discourse, grounded in nutritional science, appears to be gaining and losing ground on differing fronts. A feminist counter-discourse, which rejects the equation of health with slimness, seems to be providing women and girls with a means to repel the dominant discourse – though it is less clear that their food practices maintain such resistance. On the other hand, the equation of healthy eating with a war against obesity (Biltekoff 2013) appears to be expanding the capillary-like action of the dominant discourse, enfolding men and boys into the web of self-discipline, self-surveillance, and self-denial that is required to produce docile bodies and proper "healthy" citizens.

At the same time, feminist discourses regarding gender inequality appear to be actively undermined by messages that gendered structural constraints (as well as feminism itself) are passé at best (Everingham, Stevenson, and Warner-Smith 2007). In a post-feminist turn, Canadians tend to believe that women and men share full equality and that any constraints are individual (McPhail, Beagan, and Chapman 2012). Yet with little sign of change, the women in our study continued to manage family food practices. The extent to which they did so was striking. This pattern was particularly enabled by the discourse of healthy eating and to a lesser extent the imperative on parents (mothers) to teach children middle-class eating, the distinctions of Taste, through food. Being a good woman, a good middle-class mother, can be performed if not accomplished by serving healthy food at the family table, teaching children to develop sophisticated palates, supporting their preferences for ethical or vegetarian eating, and instructing them in gender-appropriate techniques for body maintenance. Women govern themselves and each other in this regard, in a version of "gender expectations gone underground" (Beagan et al. 2008, 667) that needs to be theorized and understood within its operating language of individual choice and health.

Indeed, the mainstream healthy eating messages enjoy such discursive power that they were wielded by virtually everyone in our study, at all levels of social hierarchies, to castigate the eating practices of the invisible "unhealthy" Other. As Michèle Lamont (2000) suggests, moral boundary work is multidirectional, with members of all socio-cultural groups constructing themselves as morally worthy compared to Others. Evidently, aspects of healthy eating are employed by all groups to distance themselves from the less virtuous. It is an effective tool of moral judgment. Perhaps because the mainstream discourse is so prevalent across classes, so undiscerning in its multidirectional boundary marking, other food-related discourses may be even more effective for demarcating symbolic capital between classes. The dominant repertoires of ethical and connoisseur cosmopolitan eating, which appear to be more emergent and are less state-supported, enable people to set themselves apart from the masses.

Lastly, though empirical research on symbolic and moral boundary work has been expanding in numerous directions (see Pachucki,

Pendergrass, and Lamont 2007), it has not focused on rural and urban places and people, particularly in connection with food practices. Participants in our study often construed rural places as idyllic but could also categorize them as backward and conservative, their inhabitants unsophisticated and uneducated. In their descriptions of rural eating practices, urban-dwellers and those who had previously lived in cities produced some of the most hostile Othering in the entire study. Interestingly, any sense of urban centres as base and immoral (Thorpe 2012) seems to have dwindled, at least where food practices are concerned. Interviewees depicted urban food environments as sophisticated, ethically superior, adventurous, and healthy. The use of food to perform such rural-urban boundary work warrants further theoretical exploration.

IMPLICATIONS FOR PRACTICE

This study also has implications for food professionals, activists, and everyday consumers. Most centrally, it demonstrates that, in multiple social and geographic locations, notions of healthy, ethical, and cosmopolitan eating are not morally or socially neutral: in fact, they are used to create and maintain deep inequitable divisions on the bases of class, place, and gender. Thus, because so much is going on beneath the surface when people engage with food, effecting changes in eating habits is typically very challenging: multiple influences are at play, myriad social messages are being conveyed, and various identity projects are at work.

Virtually all our participants seemed to understand the mainstream discourse of healthy eating (Canadian Council of Food and Nutrition 2009). Yet with greater or lesser degrees of embarrassment or guilt – and occasionally with no guilt at all – they acknowledged that it did not always guide their decisions about what and how to eat. Through their food practices, they were not merely fuelling their bodies: they were also conveying to themselves and others that they were good mothers, or strong representatives of an ethnic identity, or sophisticated urbanites. Through food, people were drawing symbolic and moral boundaries to distinguish themselves from Others. Nutrition was far from the only concern when food decisions were made.

At the same time, even if people wanted to thoroughly incorporate dominant approaches to healthy, ethical, or cosmopolitan eating, they were not all equally able to do so. Economic capital and geographic location directly and immediately affected access to particular cultural repertoires concerning food. Perhaps most significantly, poverty made it difficult to follow the dictates of healthy eating, widening chasms in health outcomes between social classes. In numerous ways, poverty also made it hard to eat with dignity in Canada. The ability to perform distinction through the dominant ethical eating repertoire was virtually non-existent for families living in poverty. In large cities, such families may be able to engage in a pragmatic mode of cosmopolitan eating, though it does not enjoy the heightened social status that attends its connoisseur counterpart. In rural areas, interest in cosmopolitan eating may be tempered by lack of access, preference for familiarity, and respect for tradition, culminating in a tentative approach that is scorned by others as conservative and unsophisticated. Wealthier rural-dwellers may be able to access exotic foods that are not locally available, "buying" their distinction by transcending local taste spaces.

Research on food inequities is commonly grounded in the assumption that there are good ways of eating (which not everyone can attain) and bad ways of eating, which are practised by marginalized groups. This binary is too simplistic. Although impoverished Canadians are clearly marginalized from high-status eating practices, all our participants used food to demarcate identities and make sense of their social worlds. To put it differently, our study has shown that occupants of all social locations employ food practices to construct their own moral worth against that of other social groups. Understanding these dynamics can aid in efforts to alter eating habits to improve individual health and/or that of the planet. For example, invoking the virtue of frugality among economically marginalized groups may encourage reduction in food packaging and the critique of processed food. It may also be helpful to recognize that there are many ways of eating ethically, that people are already making principled food choices, even if they depart from the dominant "green" ethical repertoire. People from multiple social locations already care about and engage with moral issues surrounding eating.

Although there is tremendous room for agency and choice in the realm of food, our study has convinced us that any effort to change people's eating habits must acknowledge the power of the habitus.

The dispositions and cultural repertoires developed during childhood socialization continue to shape approaches to food in profound and long-lasting ways. Change is not impossible, but it is accompanied by often invisible losses: of identity, of moral and symbolic boundaries, of virtue structures and therefore moral worth, of distinction from an Other. Change requires cultural retooling, adding new elements to repertoires, work that not everybody is prepared or able to do.

We are left with considerable ambivalence concerning the ubiquitous healthy eating discourse. We have shown that it functions to hierarchically organize the eating practices of Canadians from a range of social locations relative to the practices of others. It is a tool in the construction and maintenance of social inequities. Yet some ways of eating are more or less related to long-term physical health, so rejecting the discourse because of its implications for inequities would be unreasonable. The claimed relationship between eating practices and health, however, often far outstrips the actual evidence, revealing the healthy eating discourse to be functioning as a moral discourse implicated in governance and self-governance. For example, due to its hegemony, the body image preoccupation that has long been an expectation of femininity may be infiltrating masculinity.

At a minimum, we advise skepticism regarding the healthy eating discourse and continual awareness of its role in judging and marginalizing others to reinforce one's own social and moral position. It is inevitably implicated in the politics of class, race, nationality, ethnicity, gender, and the ideals of moral citizenship. We echo Charlotte Biltekoff (2013), who argues that all dietary advice is a social, cultural, and political construction, and should be read as such. We join her in calling for a new "dietary literacy," akin to media literacy, that would "start with the assumption that all messages are constructed and have a purpose beyond the communication of nutritional facts" (ibid., 155).

Food is not solely about nutrition, of course, but distinction. Certain food practices are continually marked as morally commendable, whereas others are depicted as morally reprehensible. These distinctions are not just about who possesses food knowledge and who does not, but are centrally about differences of class, place, ethnicity, and gender. Food practices, which feel so utterly individual, so personally grounded in tastes and preferences, are irrefutably socially marked and marking. They facilitate striving for distinction and the castigation of inferiority. The construction of the Other through judgments about food is particularly powerful because it is ostensibly innocent. We hope that this study has irrevocably challenged such innocence, demonstrating the implication of food practices in systems of social inequality.

APPENDIX 1

RESEARCH METHODS

THIS STUDY EMPLOYED qualitative social science research methods, collecting data through in-depth interviews. Families were recruited from ten Canadian communities, which are described and compared in Table 1 (page 20). As noted in the Introduction, the sites included the East and West Coasts, Central Canada, and the Prairies. They included large and small cities, as well as rural areas comprised of farms, villages, and small towns. The communities varied in terms of household income and ethnic diversity.

In each geographic location, we recruited about ten families to participate in the study – as few as nine and as many as thirteen. Families had to have lived in the local area for at least two years and had to include at least one teenager and one adult woman who was willing to be interviewed. We permitted participants to define "family" as they chose, though at least some members had to live in the same household, since we were interested in how people influenced each other. We distributed posters and advertisements about the study in local media and through classified ad websites, in grocery stores and at farmers' markets, and at laundromats and restaurants; we also asked friends, colleagues, and study participants to pass posters on to others. People who were interested contacted a researcher at the local site to learn more.

Generally, we accepted anyone who was willing to participate, as long as two family members agreed to do so. We sought some variety, especially in income levels and family structures, but more through selective recruitment than by screening out families. For example, when we had a lot of low-income families in one site, we distributed posters in high-end food stores and restaurants to try to interest higher-income families. When we had no single-mother-headed families in one site, we took posters to community centres and public libraries that provided free childcare and support programs for single mothers.

In each family, we interviewed at least one teenager (aged thirteen to nineteen years) and one adult. In three families, children about to turn thirteen wanted to be our "teen" for the family. We agreed. In four families, older or younger siblings wanted to be interviewed in addition to the main teen participants. The totals across the country are listed in the Introduction and detailed in Appendix 2. We interviewed 105 families, including 123 adults and 131 teens. In some families, more than one adult volunteered to be interviewed; more commonly, more than one teenager volunteered. As a thank you, each family was given a grocery store gift card for a hundred dollars, and each teen was given a twenty-dollar gift card for a movie or music store.

Every participant was interviewed twice. Usually, each family member was interviewed separately, but sometimes the youth in a family preferred to be interviewed together. Getting teens to talk in depth can be difficult, and we found that having two or more in an interview actually helped. They finished each other's stories, challenged each other, and prompted or reminded each other of past experiences. Many of the adult men also preferred to join their female partners for an interview, rather than being interviewed on their own. Again, this enhanced the quality and depth of the exchange. Of course, we cannot know how the presence of any given individual inhibited the forthrightness of another, but we do know that interviewing people together often seemed to spark discussion.

In the first interview, which usually lasted one to two hours, people were asked about what they and their family ate. We never revealed what other family members had said, maintaining confidentiality. This was sometimes tricky, as when people said things like "I'm sure my son told you that I always –." We would jokingly reply that comments would not be shared.

We asked people to describe a typical day's eating and whether it differed on weekends and weekdays. We asked how the family decided what to eat, including how differing taste preferences were negotiated, who cooked, cleaned, and shopped for food, and how decisions were made about what to buy. We asked about food-related conflicts in the family. We asked people to indicate what was good about how they ate, what was not so good, what healthy eating meant to them, and whether health concerns affected their eating patterns. We asked whether the way in which they ate had changed and whether they would like it to change. We asked how times of greater or lesser financial resources had affected or might affect their food practices. We asked how they balanced cost, convenience, cooking skills, and ethical concerns in deciding what to eat. We asked how their eating habits related to their childhood and their culture and community. We also asked how people in the local area typically ate, to get a sense of food patterns and cultures.

At the end of the first interview, participants were given disposable cameras and asked to take photos of foods and eating places in their homes and local community. We suggested some useful subjects, such as food they liked and didn't like, or that they considered healthy or unhealthy, places they shopped or would never shop, restaurants they patronized or would never frequent, and foods they considered treats. Some volunteered to photograph the contents of their cupboards, fridges, and freezers, and we began to suggest this to participants, if they were willing. Some people used the disposable cameras that we had given them, in which case we had the film developed prior to the second interview. Others used their own digital cameras, and we copied their photos onto USB drives.

The second interview sought more depth concerning relationships among place, gender, class, ethnicity, age, and food practices. It used two photo-elicitation methods to help reveal aspects of everyday food practices that might be so taken for granted that they were not easy to explain. These interviews began by looking through the participant's photographs, asking questions to get the person to speak about each one and what it represented. We recorded those conversations. The pictures served as a kind of visual prompt, helping people remember to tell us about specific meals, or food stores, or restaurants they might otherwise have forgotten. They gave us another entrance to the food worlds of interviewees.

At the same time, we wanted to explore food practices that caused discomfort or uncertainty. For example, those who had never eaten sushi were unlikely to provide a photo of it to tell us that they didn't eat it – unless someone else in their family ate it. But if we showed them a photo of sushi, they could tell us why they didn't like it or would never try it, helping us to understand the logic that underlay their food practices. The second photo-elicitation technique did exactly that.

We provided two sets of photographs for people to examine. The first consisted of twenty-six shots of food, including fast, fancy, and simple food, dishes from various ethnic cuisines, and vegetarian and meat-based meals. Selecting photos that presented an adequate range of food types without making the exercise too long was challenging. The images were sushi, beef Wellington, a hot dog, beautifully arranged fish and vegetables, a fast-food soft-shell taco, a bacon cheeseburger with fries, a tossed salad, chicken soup, beef stew, a grilled cheese sandwich, macaroni and cheese, butter chicken, hummus and falafel, a North Indian thali meal, pizza, an Ethiopian meal with injera bread and several dishes, pot roast, a cold soup, a Korean meal with kimchee and several other dishes, roti with curried chickpeas and dahl, tacos with rice and beans, couscous and vegetables, spaghetti with bread and red wine, a vegetarian stir-fry, white fish with rice, and a spring green salad.

We asked participants to sort the photos according to whether or not they would be comfortable eating the foods depicted. Some also created a neutral pile. Most importantly, we got them to talk about *why* they were categorizing the photos, explaining their rationales as they went. Then we did the exercise again, asking them to sort the images according to their healthiness or unhealthiness. Again, some people created a neutral pile. And again, we talked with them about why they classified foods as they did. They sorted the images again, into piles of typically men's or women's (boys' or girls') food, then again into typically adult or teen food, both times allowing a neutral pile and both times conversing about rationales. If there was time, we also asked which dishes they would be comfortable preparing themselves, to get a sense of cooking skills. This photo-sorting exercise proved very powerful, especially to uncover ways in which food familiarity or adventurousness featured differently for participants. The overlap among categories of healthy, adult, and feminine foods, and among unhealthy, teen, and masculine foods, was also fascinating.

Our second set of photos showed fifteen types of restaurants, ranging from very informal cafeterias and fast-food places to mall food courts, diners and family eateries, and pubs, buffets, and very formal restaurants. Participants sorted these photos to indicate where they would and would not feel comfortable eating. Some created a neutral pile. In discussing their categories, we wanted to understand how class background influenced an intangible sense of comfort or discomfort with particular kinds of food spaces, a sense of belonging or not belonging. We also included some ethnic diversity, such as a Chinese buffet and a Japanese restaurant, hoping to get people to talk about their degree of openness to differing eating spaces. This technique also proved particularly valuable in uncovering a sense of food omnivorousness, the willingness to eat from any cuisine and any social class – some people described clear boundaries about where they would and would not eat, and others seemed proud to state they would eat absolutely anywhere.

Verbatim transcripts of all the interviews were prepared and entered into a software program (AtlasTi) to help organize our analysis. Key photographs and field notes recording interviewer reflections on the interviews were also entered into the software. The main activities of data analysis consisted of reading and rereading transcripts, comparing one person or family with another, and later comparing patterns by gender, class, place, and ethnicity.

Early in the process, we met face-to-face, all having analyzed the same transcripts. We collectively developed a list of codes, words that we used to label themes or patterns in the data, such as "healthy eating" for comments that dealt with food practices people considered healthful. We met regularly with research assistants at each site and talked in depth about interpreting the data and applying codes. We spoke on the phone every month and discussed any questions about data or codes, and any new codes we were considering. AtlasTi allowed us to easily keep up-to-date definitions of our codes, with examples. Regular discussions were essential if our thinking about the data analysis was to remain similar across sites, and they allowed us to pay particular attention to people or issues that seemed not to fit our analyses.

When all the interviews for each family were coded, the analyst wrote a summary "family memo," recording the main themes in that family's food practices. The memos, which were three to five pages long, discussed the family's overall eating practices, its main food concerns, how it negotiated intrafamilial differences, how health and financial issues shaped its food practices, and what food was centrally about for this family. The memos helped us capture an overall sense of the family as an interactive unit.

While data analysis was under way, we categorized each household by social class, creating definitions and discussing ambiguous families until we reached consensus. We did the same to identify migration patterns and class trajectories. Finally, for each of the chapters in the book, we used the relevant family memos, reread the full transcripts, wrote new memos focused on the topic, pulled quotes from the transcripts by individual codes (such as "vegetarian") and intersections of codes ("vegetarian" and "family tensions"), created new codes and coded raw data again, and compared patterns by gender and/or migration and/or class. We talked about our emerging analyses with the team and shared theoretical insights and sources that might be helpful. We collectively identified ideal case studies to illustrate the themes of each chapter.

APPENDIX 2

STUDY PARTICIPANT DEMOGRAPHICS

Place	Kent	Vancouver	Athabasca	Edmonton	Prince Edward	Kingston	South Parkdale	North Riverdale	Kings	Halifax	Totals
Participants	n=27	n=26	n=26	n=31	n=19	n=26	n=24	n=24	n=27	n=24	n=254
Women	11	11	10	11	9	13	10	10	10	10	105
Men	3	3	3	2	0	0	1	2	2	2	18
Girls	8	4	7	11	7	7	9	5	11	8	77
Boys	5	8	6	7	3	6	4	7	4	4	54
Age											
9–12	0	0	0	1	0	2	1	0	0	0	4
13–15	8	6	9	9	8	7	7	8	7	6	75
16–19	5	6	4	7	2	4	5	4	8	6	51
20–29	0	0	0	1	0	0	0	0	0	0	1
30–39	3	1	1	3	1	3	0	0	3	1	16
40–49	6	7	8	6	7	7	7	7	6	9	70
50–60+	5	6	4	4	1	3	4	5	3	2	37

Place	Kent $n=14$	Vancouver $n=14$	Athabasca $n=13$	Edmonton $n=13$	Prince Edward $n=9$	Kingston $n=13$	South Parkdale $n=11$	North Riverdale $n=12$	Kings $n=12$	Halifax $n=12$	Totals
Education: Parents only											
Less than high school	0	0	1	0	0	0	0	1	0	1	3
High-school diploma	3	1	2	0	1	0	2	0	2	1	12
Some post-secondary	4	3	3	0	3	2	3	1	2	3	24
Undergraduate degree	4	3	4	3	3	5	2	5	2	3	34
Graduate degree	1	4	2	6	1	1	2	5	1	2	25
College diploma	0	1	0	2	1	5	2	0	4	2	17
Trade	2	2	1	2	0	0	0	0	1	0	8
Ethnicity											
Euro-Canadian	25	12	24	21	19	20	13	21	27	16	198
Aboriginal	2	7	2	0	0	2	0	0	0	2	15
South Asian	0	2	0	8	0	2	0	0	0	0	12
Chinese	0	4	0	0	0	2	0	0	0	0	6
African/African Canadian	0	0	0	0	0	0	0	0	0	4	4
Other/Mixed	0	1	0	2	0	0	11	3	0	2	19

Place	Kent n=11	Vancouver n=11	Athabasca n=10	Edmonton n=11	Prince Edward n=9	Kingston n=13	South Parkdale n=10	North Riverdale n=10	Kings n=10	Halifax n=10	Totals n=105
Social class by family											
Working poor/Impoverished	1	4	1	1	3	6	3	2	3	2	26
Working class	3	2	1	1	2	2	1	0	3	3	18
Lower middle class	6	1	3	1	2	1	4	2	2	3	25
Upper middle class	1	4	5	8	2	4	2	6	2	2	36
Income											
< 30,000	2	4	0	3	3	5	4	3	3	2	29
30–75,000	5	3	2	2	6	4	4	1	3	4	34
76–150,000	4	4	7	6	0	3	0	3	4	2	33
> 150,000	0	0	0	0	0	1	2	3	0	2	8
Not reported	0	0	1	0	0	0	0	0	0	0	1
Family structure											
Mother, father, children	10	5	8	9	6	4	5	5	7	6	65
Single mother, children	1	3	2	2	3	7	3	4	3	2	30
Multi-generational	0	3	0	0	0	2	2	1	0	2	10

WORKS CITED

Adams, Matthew, and Jayne Raisborough. 2010. "Making a Difference: Ethical Consumption and the Everyday." *British Journal of Sociology* 61 (2): 256–74. http://dx.doi.org/10.1111/j.1468-4446.2010.01312.x.

Adey, Peter. 2010. *Aerial Life: Spaces, Mobilities, Affects.* Oxford: Wiley-Blackwell. http://dx.doi.org/10.1002/9781444324631.

Anderson, Eric. 2002. "Openly Gay Athletes: Contesting Hegemonic Masculinity in a Homophobic Environment." *Gender and Society* 16 (6): 860–77. http://dx.doi.org/10.1177/089124302237892.

Appadurai, Arjun. 1996. *Modernity at Large: Cultural Dimensions of Globalization.* Minneapolis: University of Minnesota Press.

Avakian, Arlene Voski. 2005. "Shish Kebab Armenians? Food and the Construction and Maintenance of Ethnic and Gender Identities among Armenian American Feminists." In *From Betty Crocker to Feminist Food Studies: Critical Perspectives on Women and Food,* ed. Arlene Voski Avakian and Barbara Haber, 257–80. Boston: University of Massachusetts Press.

Baker, Daniel, Kelly Hamshaw, and Jane Kolodinsky. 2009. "Who Shops at the Market? Using Consumer Surveys to Grow Farmers' Markets: Findings from a Regional Market in Northwestern Vermont." *Journal of Extension* 47 (6): 1–9.

Barr, Susan I., and Gwen E. Chapman. 2002. "Perceptions and Practices of Self-Defined Current Vegetarian, Former Vegetarian and Nonvegetarian Women." *Journal of the American Dietetic Association* 102 (3): 354–60. http://dx.doi.org/10.1016/S0002-8223(02)90083-0.

Bartky, Sandra Lee. 1997. "Foucault, Femininity, and the Modernization of Patriarchal Power." In *Feminist Social Thought: A Reader,* ed. Diana T. Meyers, 93–111. New York: Routledge.

Bassett, Raewyn, Gwen E. Chapman, and Brenda L. Beagan. 2008. "Autonomy and Control: The Co-construction of Adolescent Food Choice." *Appetite* 50 (2–3): 325–32. http://dx.doi.org/10.1016/j.appet.2007.08.009.

Beagan, Brenda L., Gwen E. Chapman, Andrea D'Sylva, and B. Raewyn Bassett. 2008. "'It's Just Easier for Me to Do It': Rationalizing the Family Division of Foodwork." *Sociology* 42 (4): 653–71. http://dx.doi.org/10.1177/0038038508091621.

Beagan, Brenda L., Svetlana Ristovski-Slijepcevic, and Gwen E. Chapman. 2010. "'People Are Just Becoming More Conscious of How Everything's Connected': 'Ethical' Food Consumption in Two Regions of Canada." *Sociology* 44 (4): 751–69. http://dx.doi.org/10.1177/0038038510369364.

Beausoleil, Natalie. 2009. "An Impossible Task? Preventing Disordered Eating in the Context of the Current Obesity Panic." In *Biopolitics and the "Obesity Epidemic": Governing Bodies,* ed. Jan Wright and Valerie Harwood, 93–107. New York: Routledge.

Beausoleil, Natalie, and Pamela Ward. 2010. "Fat Panic in Canadian Public Health Policy: Obesity as Different and Unhealthy." *Radical Psychology* 8 (1). http://www.radicalpsychology.org.

Bell, Kirsten, and Darlene McNaughton. 2007. "Feminism and the Invisible Fat Man." *Body and Society* 13 (1): 107–31. http://dx.doi.org/10.1177/1357034X07074780.

Bellavance, Guy, Myrtille Valex, and Michel Ratté. 2004. "Le goût des autres: une analyse des répertoires culturels de nouvelles élites omnivores." *Sociologie et sociétés* 36 (1): 27–57. http://dx.doi.org/10.7202/009581ar.

Bennett, Tony. 2011. "Culture, Choice, Necessity: A Political Critique of Bourdieu's Aesthetic." *Poetics* 39 (6): 530–46. http://dx.doi.org/10.1016/j.poetic.2011.09.001.

Bennett, Tony, Mike Savage, Elizabeth Silva, Alan Warde, Modesto Gayo-Cal, and David Wright, eds. 2009. *Culture, Class, Distinction.* Abingdon, UK: Routledge.

Biltekoff, Charlotte. 2013. *Eating Right in America: The Cultural Politics of Food and Health.* Durham, NC: Duke University Press. http://dx.doi.org/10.1215/9780822377276.

Binnie, Jon, Julian Holloway, Steve Millington, and Craig Young, eds. 2006. *Cosmopolitan Urbanism.* London: Routledge.

Blue, Gwendolyn. 2008. "If It Ain't Alberta, It Ain't Beef: Local Food, Regional Identity, (Inter)national Politics." *Food, Culture and Society* 11 (1): 69–85. http://dx.doi.org/10.2752/155280108X276168.

Bondy, Tierney, and Vishal Talwar. 2011. "Through Thick and Thin: How Fair Trade Consumers Have Reacted to the Global Economic Recession." *Journal of Business Ethics* 101 (3): 365–83. http://dx.doi.org/10.1007/s10551-010-0726-4.

Bordo, Susan. 1993. *Unbearable Weight: Feminism, Western Culture, and the Body.* Berkeley: University of California Press.

Boult, David A. 2004. *Hunger in the Arctic: Food (In)security in Inuit Communities.* Ottawa: Ajunnginiq Centre, National Aboriginal Health Organization. http://www.naho.ca/documents/it/2004_Inuit_Food_Security.pdf.

Bourdieu, Pierre. 1984. *Distinction*. Cambridge, MA: Harvard University Press.

—. 1986. "The Forms of Capital." In *Handbook of Theory and Research for the Sociology of Education*, ed. John G. Richardson, 241–58. New York: Greenwood Press.

Brown, Elizabeth, Sandrine Dury, and Michelle Holdsworth. 2009. "Motivations of Consumers That Use Local, Organic Fruit and Vegetable Box Schemes in Central England and Southern France." *Appetite* 53 (2): 183–88. http://dx.doi.org/10.1016/j.appet.2009.06.006.

Brown, Keith R. 2009. "The Social Dynamics and Durability of Moral Boundaries." *Sociological Forum* 24 (4): 854–76. http://dx.doi.org/10.1111/j.1573-7861.2009.01139.x.

Brownlie, Douglas, and Paul Hewer. 2007. "Prime Beef Cuts: Culinary Images for Thinking 'Men.'" *Consumption Markets and Culture* 10 (3): 229–50. http://dx.doi.org/10.1080/10253860701365371.

Bruner, Mark W., Joshua Lawson, William Pickett, William Boyce, and Ian Janssen. 2008. "Rural Canadian Adolescents Are More Likely to Be Obese Compared with Urban Adolescents." *International Journal of Pediatric Obesity* 3 (4): 205–11. http://dx.doi.org/10.1080/17477160802158477.

Cairns, Kate, Josée Johnston, and Norah MacKendrick. 2013. "Feeding the 'Organic Child': Mothering Through Ethical Consumption." *Journal of Consumer Culture* 13 (2): 97–118. http://dx.doi.org/10.1177/1469540513480162.

Canadian Council of Food and Nutrition. 2009. "Tracking Nutrition Trends: A 20 Year History." http://www.cfdr.ca/Downloads/CCFN-docs/20-Years-of-TNT-%28Sep12%29-Final.aspx.

Caplan, Pat. 1997. "Approaches to the Study of Food, Health and Identity." In *Food, Health and Identity*, ed. Pat Caplan, 1–31. New York: Routledge.

Chapman, Gwen E., and Brenda L. Beagan. 2003. "Women's Perspectives on Nutrition, Health and Breast Cancer." *Journal of Nutrition Education and Behavior* 35 (3): 135–41. http://dx.doi.org/10.1016/S1499-4046(06)60197-8.

—. 2011. "Meanings of Food, Eating, and Health in Punjabi Families Living in Vancouver, Canada." *Health Education Journal* 70 (1): 102–12. http://dx.doi.org/10.1177/0017896910373031.

—. 2013. "Food Practices and Transnational Identities: Case Studies of Two Punjabi Canadian Families." *Food, Culture and Society* 16 (3): 367–86. DOI: 10.2752/175174413X13673466711688.

Charles, Nickie, and Marion Kerr. 1988. *Women, Food and Families*. Manchester, UK: Manchester University Press.

Chernin, Kim. 1985. *The Hungry Self: Women, Eating and Identity*. New York: Harper and Row.

Cherry, Elizabeth. 2006. "Veganism as a Cultural Movement: A Relational Approach." *Social Movement Studies* 5 (2): 155–70. http://dx.doi.org/10.1080/14742830600807543.

City of Toronto. 2006a. "North Riverdale Neighbourhood Profile." http://www.toronto.ca/.

—. 2006b. "South Parkdale Neighbourhood Profile." http://www.toronto.ca/.

Classen, Constance. 2005. "The Witch's Senses: Sensory Ideologies and Transgressive Femininities from the Renaissance to Modernity." In *Empire of the Senses,* ed. David Howes, 70–84. Oxford: Berg.

Clifford, James. 1997. *Routes: Travel and Translation in the Late Twentieth Century.* Cambridge, MA: Harvard University Press.

Collins, Francis Leo. 2008. "Of Kimchi and Coffee: Globalisation, Transnationalism and Familiarity in Culinary Consumption." *Social and Cultural Geography* 9 (2): 151–69. http://dx.doi.org/10.1080/14649360701856094.

Connell, R.W., and James W. Messerschmidt. 2005. "Hegemonic Masculinity: Rethinking the Concept." *Gender and Society* 19 (6): 829–59. http://dx.doi.org/10.1177/0891243205278639.

Corrigall-Brown, Catherine, and Fred Wein. 2009. "Regional Inequality." In *Social Inequality in Canada,* 5th ed., ed. Edward Grabb and Neil Guppy, 324–47. Toronto: Pearson Prentice Hall.

Coveney, J. 1998. "The Government and Ethics of Health Promotion: The Importance of Michel Foucault." *Health Education Research: Theory and Practice* 13 (3): 459–68. http://dx.doi.org/10.1093/her/13.3.459.

—. 1999. "The Science and Spirituality of Nutrition." *Critical Public Health* 9 (1): 23–37. http://dx.doi.org/10.1080/09581599908409217.

—. 2000. *Food, Morals and Meaning: The Pleasure and Anxiety of Eating.* London: Routledge.

Crawford, Robert. 2006. "Health as a Meaningful Social Practice." *Health* 10 (4): 401–20.

Creed, Gerald W., and Barbara Ching. 1997. "Recognizing Rusticity: Identity and the Power of Place." In *Knowing Your Place: Rural Identity and Cultural Identity,* ed. Barbara Ching and Gerald W. Creed, 1–39. New York: Routledge.

Cresswell, Tim, and Peter Merriman, eds. 2011. *Geographies of Mobilities: Practices, Spaces, Subjects.* Burlington, VT: Ashgate.

Das Gupta, Monisha. 1997. "'What Is Indian about You?': A Gendered, Transnational Approach to Ethnicity." *Gender and Society* 11 (5): 572–96. http://dx.doi.org/10.1177/089124397011005004.

de Souza, Paula, and Karen Ciclitira. 2005. "Men and Dieting: A Qualitative Analysis." *Journal of Health Psychology* 10 (6): 793–804.

Desjarlais, Robert R. 1992. *Body and Emotion: The Aesthetics of Illness and Healing in the Nepal Himalayas.* Philadelphia: University of Pennsylvania Press.

DeSoucey, Michaela. 2010. "Gastronationalism: Food Traditions and Authenticity Politics in the European Union." *American Sociological Review* 75 (3): 432–55. http://dx.doi.org/10.1177/0003122410372226.

Devadason, Ranji. 2010. "Cosmopolitanism, Geographical Imaginaries and Belonging in North London." *Urban Studies* (Edinburgh, Scotland) 47 (14): 2945–63. http://dx.doi.org/10.1177/0042098009360228.

DeVault, Marjorie L. 1991. *Feeding the Family.* Chicago: University of Chicago Press.

Douglas, Mary. 1966. *Purity and Danger: An Analysis of Concepts of Pollution and Taboo.* London: Routledge and Kegan Paul. http://dx.doi.org/10.4324/9780203361832.

D'Sylva, Andrea, and Brenda L. Beagan. 2011. "'Food Is Culture, but It's Also Power': The Role of Food in Ethnic and Gender Identity Construction among Goan Canadian Women." *Journal of Gender Studies* 20 (3): 279–89. http://dx.doi.org/10.1080/09589236.2011.593326.

Duruz, Jean. 2005. "Eating at the Borders: Culinary Journeys." *Environment and Planning D: Society and Space* 23 (1): 51–69. http://dx.doi.org/10.1068/d52j.

Ellaway, Anne, and Sally Macintyre. 2000. "Shopping for Food in Socially Contrasting Localities." *British Food Journal* 102 (1): 52–59. http://dx.doi.org/10.1108/00070700010310632.

Everett, Holly. 2009. "Vernacular Health Moralities and Culinary Tourism in Newfoundland and Labrador." *Journal of American Folklore* 122 (483): 28–52. http://dx.doi.org/10.1353/jaf.0.0048.

Everingham, Christine, Deborah Stevenson, and Penny Warner-Smith. 2007. "'Things Are Getting Better All the Time'? Challenging the Narrative of Women's Progress from a Generational Perspective." *Sociology* 41 (3): 419–37. http://dx.doi.org/10.1177/0038038507076615.

Ferguson, Hilary. 2011. "Inuit Food (In)security in Canada: Assessing the Implications and Effectiveness of Policy." *Queen's Policy Review* 2 (2): 54–79.

Flegal, Katherine M., Barry I. Graubard, David F. Williamson, and Mitchell H. Gail. 2007. "Cause-Specific Excess Deaths Associated with Underweight, Overweight, and Obesity." *Journal of the American Medical Association* 298 (17): 2028–37. http://dx.doi.org/10.1001/jama.298.17.2028.

Food Secure Canada. 2014. "Who We Are." http://foodsecurecanada.org.

Foucault, Michel. 1979. *Discipline and Punish: The Birth of the Prison.* Trans. Alan Sheridan. New York: Random House.

—. 1980. *Power/Knowledge: Selected Interviews and Other Writings, 1972–1977.* New York: Pantheon.

—. 1988. "Technologies of the Self." In *Technologies of the Self: A Seminar with Michel Foucault,* ed. Luther H. Martin, Huck Gutman, and Patrick H. Hutton, 16–49. Amherst: University of Massachusetts Press.

—. 1991. "Governmentality." In *The Foucault Effect: Studies in Governmentality with Two Lectures by and an Interview with Michel Foucault,* ed. Graham Burchell, Colin Gordon, and Peter Miller, 87–104. Chicago: University of Chicago Press.

Fox, Nick, and Katie J. Ward. 2008. "You Are What You Eat? Vegetarianism, Health and Identity." *Social Science and Medicine* 66 (12): 2585–95. http://dx.doi.org/10.1016/j.socscimed.2008.02.011.

Garriguet, Didier. 2006. *Nutrition: Findings from the Canadian Community Health Survey: Overview of Canadians' Eating Habits, 2004.* Ottawa: Statistics Canada, Health Statistics Division. http://publications.gc.ca/collections/Collection/Statcan/82-620-M/82-620-MIE2006002.pdf.

Giddens, Anthony. 1984. *The Constitution of Society: Outline of the Theory of Structuration.* Cambridge: Polity Press.

Gilbert, Dennis L. 2008. *The American Class Structure in an Age of Growing Inequality.* London: Sage.

Gilliom, John. 2001. *Overseers of the Poor: Surveillance, Resistance, and the Limits of Privacy.* Chicago: University of Chicago Press.

Gilman, Sander L. 2004. *Fat Boys: A Slim Book.* Lincoln: University of Nebraska Press.

Gossard, Marcia Hill, and Richard York. 2003. "Social Structure Influences on Meat Consumption." *Human Ecology Review* 10 (1): 1–9.

Gough, Brendan. 2007. "'Real Men Don't Diet': An Analysis of Contemporary Newspaper Representations of Men, Food and Health." *Social Science and Medicine* 64 (2): 326–37. http://dx.doi.org/10.1016/j.socscimed.2006.09.011.

Gough, Brendan, and Mark T. Conner. 2006. "Barriers to Healthy Eating amongst Men: A Qualitative Analysis." *Social Science and Medicine* 62 (2): 387–95. http://dx.doi.org/10.1016/j.socscimed.2005.05.032.

Greene-Finestone, L.S., M.K. Campbell, S.E. Evers, and I.A. Gutmanis. 2008. "Attitudes and Health Behaviours of Young Adolescent Omnivores and Vegetarians: A School-Based Study." *Appetite* 51 (1): 104–10. http://dx.doi.org/10.1016/j.appet.2007.12.005.

Griffith, R. Marie. 2004. *Born Again Bodies: Flesh and Spirit in American Christianity.* Berkeley: University of California Press.

Grosz, Elizabeth. 1994. *Volatile Bodies: Toward a Corporeal Feminism.* Bloomington: Indiana University Press.

Guthman, Julie. 2003. "Fast Food/Organic Food: Reflexive Tastes and the Making of 'Yuppie Chow.'" *Social and Cultural Geography* 4 (1): 45–58. http://dx.doi.org/10.1080/1464936032000049306.

—. 2008. "'If They Only Knew': Color Blindness and Universalism in California Alternative Food Institutions." *Professional Geographer* 60 (3): 387–97. http://dx.doi.org/10.1080/00330120802013679.

Halkier, Bente. 2009. "Suitable Cooking? Performances and Positionings in Cooking Practices among Danish Women." *Food, Culture and Society* 12 (3): 357–77. http://dx.doi.org/10.2752/175174409X432030.

Hannerz, Ulf. 1996. *Transnational Connections.* London: Routledge.

Harris, R. Cole. 2012. "Regionalism." In *The Canadian Encyclopedia.* http://www.thecanadianencyclopedia.com/en/article/regionalism/.

Hashimoto, Atsuko, and David J. Telfer. 2006. "Selling Canadian Culinary Tourism: Branding the Global and the Regional Product." *Tourism Geographies: An International Journal of Tourism Space, Place and Environment* 8 (1): 31–55. http://dx.doi.org/10.1080/14616680500392465.

Hay, M. Cameron. 2008. "Reading Sensations: Understanding the Process of Distinguishing 'Fine' from 'Sick.'" *Transcultural Psychiatry* 45 (2): 198–229. http://dx.doi.org/10.1177/1363461508089765.

Health Canada. 2007. "Canada's Food Guides from 1942 to 1992." http://www.hc-sc.gc.ca/fn-an/food-guide-aliment/context/fg_history-histoire_ga-eng.php.

Heldke, Lisa. 2003. *Exotic Appetites: Ruminations of a Food Adventurer.* New York: Routledge.

Hillier, Harry H. 1996. *Canadian Society: A Macro Analysis.* Scarborough: Prentice Hall Canada.

hooks, bell. 1992. "Eating the Other: Desire and Resistance." In *Black Looks: Race and Representation,* 21–39. Boston: South End Press.

Human Resources and Skills Development Canada. 2013. "Canadians in Context — Geographic Distribution." http://www4.hrsdc.gc.ca/.3ndic.1t.4r@ -eng.jsp?iid=34Q1.

Ismailov, Rovshan M., and Scott T. Leatherdale. 2010. "Rural-Urban Differences in Overweight and Obesity among a Large Sample of Adolescents in Ontario." *International Journal of Pediatric Obesity* 5 (4): 351–60. http://dx. doi.org/10.3109/17477160903449994.

Johnston, Carol S., Christopher A. Taylor, and Jeffery S. Hampl. 2000. "More Americans Are Eating '5 a Day' but Intakes of Dark Green and Cruciferous Vegetables Remain Low." *Journal of Nutrition* 130 (12): 3063–67.

Johnston, Josée. 2008. "The Citizen-Consumer Hybrid: Ideological Tensions and the Case of Whole Foods Market." *Theory and Society* 37 (3): 229–70. http://dx.doi.org/10.1007/s11186-007-9058-5.

Johnston, Josée, and Shyon Baumann. 2010. *Foodies: Democracy and Distinction in the Gourmet Foodscape.* New York: Routledge.

Johnston, Josée, Shyon Baumann, and Kate Cairns. 2009. "The National and the Cosmopolitan in Cuisine: Constructing America through Gourmet Food Writing." In *The Globalization of Food,* ed. David Inglis and Debra Gimlin, 161–84. Oxford: Berg.

Johnston, Josée, Alexandra Rodney, and Michelle Szabo. 2012. "Place, Ethics, and Everyday Eating: A Tale of Two Neighbourhoods." *Sociology* 46 (6): 1091–108. http://dx.doi.org/10.1177/0038038511435060.

Johnston, Josée, Michelle Szabo, and Alexandra Rodney. 2011. "Good Food, Good People: Understanding the Cultural Repertoire of Ethical Eating." *Journal of Consumer Culture* 11 (3): 293–318. http://dx.doi.org/10.1177/ 1469540511417996.

Kaufmann, Vincent, Manfred Max Bergman, and Dominique Joye. 2004. "Motility: Mobility as Capital." *International Journal of Urban and Regional Research* 28 (4): 745–56. http://dx.doi.org/10.1111/j.0309-1317.2004.00549.x.

Kaufmann, Vincent, and Bertrand Montulet. 2008. "Between Social and Spatial Mobilities: The Issue of Social Fluidity." In *Tracing Mobilities: Towards a Cosmopolitan Perspective,* ed. Weert Canzler, Vincent Kaufmann, and Sven Kesselring, 37–56. Burlington, VT: Ashgate.

Kenneally, Rhona Richman. 2009. "'There *Is* a Canadian Cuisine, and It Is Unique in All the World': Crafting National Food Culture during the Long 1960s." In *What's to Eat? Entrées in Canadian Food History,* ed. Nathalie Cooke, 167–96. Montreal and Kingston: McGill-Queen's University Press.

Kent, Le'a. 2001. "Fighting Abjection: Representing Fat Women." In *Bodies Out of Bounds,* ed. Jana Evans Braziel and Kathleen LeBesco, 130–52. Berkeley: University of California Press.

Kirkey, Sharon. 2008. "Canadian Men More Likely to Be Obese." *Ottawa Citizen.com.* http://www2.canada.com/ottawacitizen/health/story.html?id= bada7d12-8a87-4962-9509-a94754bbddac&p=1.

Korsmeyer, Carolyn. 1999. *Making Sense of Taste*. Ithaca: Cornell University Press.

Lacobbo, Karen, and Michael Lacobbo. 2006. *Vegetarians and Vegans in America Today*. Westport, CT: Praeger.

Lamont, Michèle. 1992. *Money, Morals, and Manners: The Culture of the French and the American Upper-Middle Class*. Chicago: University of Chicago Press. http://dx.doi.org/10.7208/chicago/9780226922591.001.0001.

—. 2000. *The Dignity of Working Men: Morality and the Boundaries of Race, Class and Immigration*. Cambridge, MA: Harvard University Press.

—. 2010. "Looking Back at Bourdieu." In *Cultural Analysis and Bourdieu's Legacy: Settling Accounts and Developing Alternatives,* ed. Elizabeth Silva and Alan Warde, 128–41. London: Routledge.

Lamont, Michèle, and Sada Aksartova. 2002. "Ordinary Cosmopolitanisms: Strategies for Bridging Racial Boundaries among Working-Class Men." *Theory, Culture and Society* 19 (4): 1–25. http://dx.doi.org/10.1177/0263276402019004001.

Lamont, Michèle, and Virag Molnár. 2002. "The Study of Boundaries in the Social Sciences." *Annual Review of Sociology* 28 (1): 167–95. http://dx.doi.org/10.1146/annurev.soc.28.110601.141107.

Lareau, Annette. 2002. "Invisible Inequality: Social Class and Childrearing in Black Families and White Families." *American Sociological Review* 67 (5): 747–76. http://dx.doi.org/10.2307/3088916.

—. 2011. *Unequal Childhoods: Class, Race and Family Life*. Berkeley: University of California Press.

Lawler, Steph. 1999. "'Getting Out and Getting Away': Women's Narratives of Class Mobility." *Feminist Review* 63 (1): 3–24. http://dx.doi.org/10.1080/014177899339036.

—. 2005. "Disgusted Subjects: The Making of Middle-Class Identities." *Sociological Review* 53 (3): 429–46. http://dx.doi.org/10.1111/j.1467-954X.2005.00560.x.

Lawton, Julia, Naureen Ahmad, Lisa Hanna, Margaret Douglas, Harpreet Bains, and Nina Hallowell. 2008. "'We Should Change Ourselves, but We Can't': Accounts of Food and Eating Practices amongst British Pakistanis and Indians with Type 2 Diabetes." *Ethnicity and Health* 13 (4): 305–19. http://dx.doi.org/10.1080/13557850701882910.

Lee, Jo, and Tim Ingold. 2006. "Fieldwork on Foot: Perceiving, Routing and Socializing." In *Locating the Field: Space, Place and Context in Anthropology,* ed. Simon Coleman and Peter Collins, 67–86. Oxford: Berg.

Liese, Angela D., Kristina E. Weis, Delores Pluto, Emily Smith, and Andrew Lawson. 2007. "Food Store Types, Availability, and Cost of Foods in a Rural Environment." *Journal of the American Dietetic Association* 107 (11): 1916–23. http://dx.doi.org/10.1016/j.jada.2007.08.012.

Little, Jo, Brian Ilbery, and David Watts. 2009. "Gender, Consumption and the Relocalisation of Food: A Research Agenda." *Sociologia Ruralis* 49 (3): 201–17. http://dx.doi.org/10.1111/j.1467-9523.2009.00492.x.

Lupton, Deborah. 1996. *Food, the Body and the Self*. London: Sage.

—. 2001. "The Heart of the Meal: Food Preferences and Habits among Rural Australian Couples." *Sociology of Health and Illness* 22 (1): 94–109.

Lyons, Antonia C. 2009. "Masculinities, Femininities, Behaviour and Health." *Social and Personality Psychology Compass* 3 (4): 394–412. http://dx.doi.org/ 10.1111/j.1751-9004.2009.00192.x.

Macionis, John J., and Linda M. Gerber. 2011. *Sociology.* 7th Canadian ed. Toronto: Pearson.

Mankekar, Purnima. 2005. "'India Shopping': Indian Grocery Stores and Transnational Configurations of Belonging." In *The Cultural Politics of Food and Eating,* ed. James L. Watson and Melissa L. Caldwell, 197–214. Malden, MA: Blackwell.

Marshall, Gordon. 1998. "Goldthorpe Class Scheme." *A Dictionary of Sociology.* http://www.encyclopedia.com/doc/1O88-Goldthorpeclassscheme.html.

Martin, Debbie. 2011. "'Now We Got Lots to Eat and They're Telling Us Not to Eat It': Understanding Changes to South-east Labrador Inuit Relationships to Food." *International Journal of Circumpolar Health* 70 (4): 384–95. http:// dx.doi.org/10.3402/ijch.v70i4.17842.

McGillivray, Brett. 2010. *Canada: A Nation of Regions.* 2nd ed. Don Mills: Oxford University Press.

McPhail, Deborah. 2009. "What to Do with the 'Tubby Hubby'? 'Obesity,' the Crisis of Masculinity, and the Nuclear Family in Early Cold War Canada." *Antipode* 41 (5): 1021–50. http://dx.doi.org/10.1111/j.1467-8330.2009.00708.x.

McPhail, Deborah, Brenda L. Beagan, and Gwen E. Chapman. 2012. "'I Don't Really Want to Be Sexist but …': Denying and Re-Inscribing Gender through Food." *Food, Culture and Society* 15 (3): 473–89.

McPhail, Deborah, Gwen E. Chapman, and Brenda L. Beagan. 2011. "'Too Much of That Stuff Can't Be Good': Canadian Teens, Morality, and Fast Food Consumption." *Social Science and Medicine* 73 (2): 301–7. http://dx.doi. org/10.1016/j.socscimed.2011.05.022.

—. 2013. "The Rural and the Rotund? A Critical Interpretation of Food Deserts and Rural Adolescent Obesity in the Canadian Context." *Health and Place* 22: 132–39. http://dx.doi.org/10.1016/j.healthplace.2013.03.009.

Menzies, Kenneth, and Judy Sheeshka. 2012. "The Process of Exiting Vegetarianism: An Exploratory Study." *Canadian Journal of Dietetic Practice and Research* 73 (4): 163–68. http://dx.doi.org/10.3148/73.4.2012.163.

Merriman, Ben. 2010. "Gender Differences in Family and Peer Reaction to the Adoption of a Vegetarian Diet." *Feminism and Psychology* 20 (3): 420–27.

Mitura, Verna, and Ray Bollman. 2004. "Health Status and Behaviours of Canada's Youth: A Rural-Urban Comparison." *Rural and Small Town Canada Analysis Bulletin* 5 (3). http://www.statcan.gc.ca/pub/21-006-x/21-006-x2003003 -eng.pdf.

Monaghan, Lee F. 2008. *Men and the War on Obesity: A Sociological Study.* New York: Routledge.

Moore, Ellen E. 2008. "Raising the Bar: The Complicated Consumption of Chocolate." In *Food for Thought: Essays on Eating and Culture,* ed. Lawrence C. Rubin, 67–82. Jefferson, NC: McFarland.

Moore, Latetia V., and Ana V. Diez Roux. 2006. "Associations of Neighborhood Characteristics with the Location and Type of Food Stores." *American Journal of Public Health* 96 (2): 325–31. http://dx.doi.org/10.2105/AJPH.2004.058040.

Morgan, Kevin. 2010. "Local and Green, Global and Fair: The Ethical Food-scape and the Politics of Care." *Environment and Planning A* 42 (8): 1852–67. http://dx.doi.org/10.1068/a42364.

Mróz, Lawrence William, Gwen E. Chapman, John L. Oliffe, and Joan L. Bottorff. 2011a. "Gender Relations, Prostate Cancer and Diet: Re-Inscribing Hetero-Normative Food Practices." *Social Science and Medicine* 72 (9): 1499–506. http://dx.doi.org/10.1016/j.socscimed.2011.03.012.

—. 2011b. "Men, Food and Prostate Cancer: Gender Influences on Men's Diets." *American Journal of Men's Health* 5 (2): 177–87. http://dx.doi.org/10.1177/1557988310379152.

Narayan, Uma. 1997. *Dislocating Cultures.* New York: Routledge.

Norman, Moss E. 2011. "Embodying the Double-Bind of Masculinity: Young Men and Discourses of Normalcy, Health, Heterosexuality and Individualism." *Men and Masculinities* 14 (4): 430–49. http://dx.doi.org/10.1177/1097184X11409360.

—. 2013. "'Dere's Not Just One Kind of Fat': Embodying the 'Skinny'-Self through Constructions of the Fat Masculine Other." *Men and Masculinities* 16 (4): 407–31. http://dx.doi.org/10.1177/1097184X13502662.

O'Doherty Jensen, Katherine, and Lotte Holm. 1999. "Preferences, Quantities and Concerns: Socio-Cultural Perspectives on the Gendered Consumption of Foods." *European Journal of Clinical Nutrition* 53 (5): 351–59. http://dx.doi.org/10.1038/sj.ejcn.1600767.

Ollivier, Michèle. 2008. "Modes of Openness to Cultural Diversity: Humanist, Populist, Practical, and Indifferent." *Poetics* 36 (2–3): 120–47. http://dx.doi.org/10.1016/j.poetic.2008.02.005.

Oluwabamide, Abiodun J., and Nseabasi S. Akpan. 2010. "Environmental and Cultural Dynamics in Nutrition: A Comparison of Food Patterns in Two Nigerian Societies." *Anthropologist* 12 (2): 95–98.

Ong, Aihwa. 1999. *Flexible Citizenship: The Cultural Logics of Transnationality.* Durham, NC: Duke University Press.

Pachucki, Mark A., Sabrina Pendergrass, and Michéle Lamont. 2007. "Boundary Processes: Recent Theoretical Developments and New Contributions." *Poetics* 35 (6): 331–51. http://dx.doi.org/10.1016/j.poetic.2007.10.001.

Pandi, George. 2008. "Let's Eat Canadian, but Is There Really a National Dish?" *Canwest News Service,* 18 November. http://www.canada.com/montrealgazette/columnists/story.html?id=6ad83058-3f7b-4403-8aa8-dce47b16884e.

Perry, Cheryl L., Maureen T. Mcguire, Dianne Neumark-Sztainer, and Mary Story. 2001. "Characteristics of Vegetarian Adolescents in a Multiethnic Urban Population." *Journal of Adolescent Health* 29 (6): 406–16. http://dx.doi.org/10.1016/S1054-139X(01)00258-0.

Peterson, Richard A., and Roger M. Kern. 1996. "Changing Highbrow Taste: From Snob to Omnivore." *American Sociological Review* 61 (5): 900–7. http://dx.doi.org/10.2307/2096460.

Plotnikoff, Ronald C., Kim Bercovitz, and Constantinos A. Loucaides. 2004. "Physical Activity, Smoking, and Obesity among Canadian School Youth: Comparison between Urban and Rural Schools." *Canadian Journal of Public Health* 95 (6): 413–18.

Popkin, Barry M., Kiyah Duffey, and Penny Gordon-Larsen. 2005. "Environmental Influences on Food Choice, Physical Activity and Energy Balance." *Physiology and Behavior* 86 (5): 603–13. http://dx.doi.org/10.1016/j.physbeh.2005.08.051.

Power, Elaine M. 2003. "De-Centering the Text: Exploring the Potential for Visual Methods in the Sociology of Food." *Journal for the Study of Food and Society* 6 (2): 9–20. http://dx.doi.org/10.2752/152897903786769670.

—. 2005. "The Determinants of Healthy Eating among Low-Income Canadians." *Canadian Journal of Public Health* 96 (S3): S37–S42.

—. Forthcoming. "Governing the Child's Body: The Obesity Epidemic and (Mother) Parents' Duties in Neoliberal Consumer Society." In *Neoliberal Governance and Health: Duties, Risks and Vulnerabilities,* ed. Jessica Polzer and Elaine Power. Montreal and Kingston: McGill-Queen's University Press.

Prättälä, Ritva, Lauren Paalanen, Daiga Grinberga, Ville Helasoja, Anu Kasmel, and Janina Petkeviciene. 2007. "Gender Differences in the Consumption of Meat, Fruit and Vegetables Are Similar in Finland and the Baltic Countries." *European Journal of Public Health* 17 (5): 520–25. http://www.ncbi.nlm.nih.gov/.

Public Health Agency of Canada and the Canadian Institute for Health Information. 2011. *Obesity in Canada: A Joint Report.* Ottawa: Her Majesty the Queen in Right of Canada. http://www.phac-aspc.gc.ca/hp-ps/hl-mvs/oic-oac/assets/pdf/oic-oac-eng.pdf.

Pugh, Allison J. 2011. "Distinction, Boundaries or Bridges? Children, Inequality and the Uses of Consumer Culture." *Poetics* 39 (1): 1–18. http://dx.doi.org/10.1016/j.poetic.2010.10.002.

Raine, Kim D. 2005. "Determinants of Healthy Eating in Canada: An Overview and Synthesis." *Canadian Journal of Public Health* 96 (S3): S8–S14.

Ray, Krishnendu. 2004. *The Migrant's Table: Meals and Memories in Bengali-American Households.* Philadelphia: Temple University Press.

Rice, Carla. 2007. "Becoming the Fat Girl: Acquisition of an Unfit Identity." *Women's Studies International Forum* 30 (2): 158–74. http://dx.doi.org/10.1016/j.wsif.2007.01.001.

Rimal, Arbindra P. 2002. "Factors Affecting Meat Preferences among American Consumers." *Family Economics and Nutrition Review* 14 (2): 36–43.

Ristovski-Slijepcevic, Svetlana, Gwen E. Chapman, and Brenda L. Beagan. 2008. "Engaging with Healthy Eating Discourse(s): Ways of Knowing about Food and Health in Three Ethnocultural Groups in Canada." *Appetite* 50 (1): 167–78. http://dx.doi.org/10.1016/j.appet.2007.07.001.

—. 2010. "Being a 'Good Mother': Dietary Governmentality in the Family Food Practices of Three Ethnocultural Groups in Canada." *Health* 14 (5): 467–83.

Roth, LuAnne K. 2005. "'Beef, It's What's for Dinner': Vegetarians, Meat-Eaters and the Negotiation of Familial Relationships." *Food, Culture and Society* 8 (2): 181–200.

Ruby, Matthew B. 2012. "Vegetarianism. A Blossoming Field of Study." *Appetite* 58 (1): 141–50. http://dx.doi.org/10.1016/j.appet.2011.09.019.

Said, Edward. 1978. *Orientalism*. New York: Pantheon Books.

Sassatelli, Roberta. 2006. "Virtue, Responsibility and Consumer Choice: Framing Critical Consumerism." In *Consuming Cultures, Global Perspectives: Historical Trajectories, Transnational Exchanges,* ed. John Brewer and Frank Trentmann, 219–50. Oxford: Berg.

Sassatelli, Roberta, and Frederica Davolio. 2010. "Consumption, Pleasure and Politics: Slow Food and the Politico-Aesthetic Problematization of Food." *Journal of Consumer Culture* 10 (2): 202–32. http://dx.doi.org/10.1177/14695 40510364591.

Satia-Abouta, Jessie, Ruth E. Patterson, Alan R. Kristal, Chong Teh, and Shin-Ping Tu. 2002. "Psychosocial Predictors of Diet and Acculturation in Chinese American and Chinese Canadian Women." *Ethnicity and Health* 7 (1): 21–39. http://dx.doi.org/10.1080/13557850220146975.

Schwartz, Joel. 2000. *Fighting Poverty with Virtue: Moral Reform and America's Urban Poor, 1825–2000.* Bloomington: Indiana University Press.

Sellaeg, Kari, and Gwen E. Chapman. 2008. "Masculinity and Food Ideals of Men Who Live Alone." *Appetite* 51 (1): 120–28. http://dx.doi.org/10.1016/j.appet.2008.01.003.

Seremetakis, Nadia C. 1994. *The Senses Still*. Chicago: University of Chicago Press.

Sheller, Mimi. 2004. "Automotive Emotions: Feeling the Car." *Theory, Culture and Society* 21 (4–5): 221–42. http://dx.doi.org/10.1177/0263276404046068.

—. 2011. "Mobility." *Sociopedia.isa*. http://www.sagepub.net/isa/resources/pdf/Mobility.pdf.

Sheller, Mimi, and John Urry. 2006. "The New Mobilities Paradigm." *Environment and Planning A* 38 (2): 207–26. http://dx.doi.org/10.1068/a37268.

Shields, Margot, and Michael Tjepkema. 2006. "Regional Differences in Obesity." *Health Reports* 17 (3): 61–67.

Silva, Elizabeth, and Alan Warde, eds. 2010. *Cultural Analysis and Bourdieu's Legacy: Settling Accounts and Developing Alternatives.* Abingdon, UK: Routledge.

Silva, Elizabeth, Alan Warde, and David Wright. 2009. "Using Mixed Methods for Analysing Culture: The Cultural Capital and Social Exclusion Project." *Cultural Sociology* 3 (2): 299–316. http://dx.doi.org/10.1177/1749975509105536.

Smith, Chery, and Lois W. Morton. 2009. "Rural Food Deserts: Low-Income Perspectives on Food Access in Minnesota and Iowa." *Journal of Nutrition Education and Behavior* 41 (3): 176–87. http://dx.doi.org/10.1016/j.jneb.2008.06.008.

Sobal, Jeffrey. 2005. "Men, Meat and Marriage: Models of Masculinity." *Food and Foodways* 13 (1–2): 135–58. http://dx.doi.org/10.1080/07409710590 915409.

Statistics Canada. 2011. "2006 Community Profiles." http://www12.statcan.ca/census-recensement/2006/dp-pd/prof/92-591/index.cfm?Lang=E.

—. 2012. "Summary Tables." http://www.statcan.gc.ca/tables-tableaux/sum-som/l01/cst01/famil107a-eng.htm.

—. 2013. "Low Income Lines, 2010-2011." http://www.statcan.gc.ca/pub/75f0002m/75f0002m2012002-eng.htm.

Swidler, Ann. 1986. "Culture in Action: Symbols and Strategies." *American Sociological Review* 51 (2): 273–86. http://dx.doi.org/10.2307/2095521.

—. 2001. *Talk of Love: How Culture Matters.* Chicago: University of Chicago Press.

Taylor, Jennifer P., Susan Evers, and Mary McKenna. 2005. "Determinants of Healthy Eating in Children and Youth." *Canadian Journal of Public Health* 96 (S3): S20–S26.

Thomas, Helen, and Jamilah Ahmed. 2004. "Introduction." In *Cultural Bodies: Ethnography and Theory,* ed. Helen Thomas and Jamilah Ahmed, 1–24. Malden, MA: Blackwell. http://dx.doi.org/10.1002/9780470775837.ch.

Thorpe, Jocelyn. 2012. *Temagami's Tangled Wild: Race, Gender, and the Making of Canadian Nature.* Vancouver: UBC Press.

Thorsted, Stine, and Terese Anving. 2010. "Feeding Ideals and the Work of Feeding in Swedish Families: Interactions between Mothers and Children around the Dinner Table." *Food, Culture and Society* 13 (1): 29–46. http://dx.doi.org/10.2752/175174410X12549021368027.

Thrift, Nigel. 2004. "Movement-Space: The Changing Domain of Thinking Resulting from the Development of New Kinds of Spatial Awareness." *Economy and Society* 33 (4): 582–604. http://dx.doi.org/10.1080/0308514042000285305.

Throop, C. Jason. 2008. "From Pain to Virtue: Dysphoric Sensations and Moral Sensibilities in Yap (Waqab), Federated States of Micronesia." *Transcultural Psychiatry* 45 (2): 253–86. http://dx.doi.org/10.1177/1363461508089767.

Tilly, Charles. 1993. "Contentious Repertoire in Great Britain, 1758–1834." *Social Science History* 17 (2): 253–79. http://dx.doi.org/10.2307/1171282.

Trubek, Amy B. 2008. *The Taste of Place.* Berkeley: University of California Press.

Tye, Diane. 2008. "A Poor Man's Meal: Molasses in Atlantic Canada." *Food, Culture and Society* 11 (1): 336–53.

Urry, John. 2007. *Mobilities.* London: Polity.

Vaisey, Stephen. 2008. "Socrates, Skinner, and Aristotle: Three Ways of Thinking about Culture in Action." *Sociological Forum* 23 (3): 603–13. http://dx.doi.org/10.1111/j.1573-7861.2008.00079.x.

Vallianatos, Helen, and Kim Raine. 2008. "Consuming Food and Constructing Identities among Arabic and South Asian Immigrant Women." *Food, Culture and Society* 11 (3): 355–73. http://dx.doi.org/10.2752/175174408X347900.

Varghese, Suja, and Robin Moore-Orr. 2002. "Dietary Acculturation and Health-Related Issues of Indian Immigrant Families in Newfoundland." *Canadian Journal of Dietetic Practice and Research* 63 (2): 72–79. http://dx.doi.org/10.3148/63.2.2002.72.

Vinge, Louise. 2009. "The Five Senses in Classical Science and Ethics." In *The Sixth Sense Reader,* ed. David Howes, 107-18. Oxford: Berg.

Wandel, Margareta, and Gun Roos. 2005. "Work, Food and Physical Activity: A Qualitative Study of Coping Strategies among Men in Three Occupations." *Appetite* 44 (1): 93–102. http://dx.doi.org/10.1016/j.appet.2004.08.002.

Warde, Alan. 1997. *Consumption, Food, and Taste*. Thousand Oaks, CA: Sage.

—. 2005. "Consumption and Theories of Practice." *Journal of Consumer Culture* 5 (2): 131–53. http://dx.doi.org/10.1177/1469540505053090.

Weedon, Chris. 1987. *Feminist Practice and Poststructuralist Theory*. Oxford: Basil Blackwell.

Wolf, Naomi. 1992. *The Beauty Myth: How Images of Beauty Are Used against Women*. New York: Doubleday.

Young, Iris Marion. 2005. *On Female Body Experience: "Throwing Like a Girl" and Other Essays*. New York: Oxford University Press. http://dx.doi.org/10.1093/0195161920.001.0001.

INDEX

Note: "(t)" after a page number indicates a table.

families: definition of, 21; food in the
formation of, 4, 5, 18, 215; food-
related tensions within, 99-100,
103, 106-10, 115, 116-20, 187, 195,
214-15, 223-16
farmers' and farm markets: community building at, 68; as expensive or
pretentious, 70, 71, 140; as form of
resistance to capitalist economy,
215; sites of pleasure, 148-49;
transparency of agricultural inputs,
173
farms: access to, 163, 172, 176, 177;
factory farming, 67-68; habitus,
210; local loyalties ethos and, 75-
76, 232; meat-and-potatoes associated with, 92, 146; unhealthy
eating associated with, 183
fast foods: as cosmopolitan foods,
172; in Othering discourses, 152,
153; as unhealthy, 5, 34, 47, 153,
158, 224; as unsophisticated, 218
fast-food restaurants: cosmopolitanism
of, 27-28; markers of high social
status, 194; in study design, 22,
252
fathers: healthy eating enforced by,
54, 86, 88; on teen vegetarianism,
103; transmit sense of taste to
sons, 220; as study participants,
224
femininity: dieting and, 130; fat and,
120-23, 221, 230; of foods, 48, 49;
of vegetarian eating, 102-3. *See also*
gender; masculinity; women and
girls
First Nations, 26, 154-55, 174-75
fish and seafood, 176-77, 183
Food Guide, Canada's, 34, 40, 101,
181
food movements, 8, 239-40
food security, 68, 74-75
food shopping, 144-46, 148-50
foodie culture, 157-58
foodscapes: multicultural, 80, 89,
90-91, 171, 192, 216, 234; rural,

75-76, 168; as sites of surveillance,
46; urban, 71, 90-91, 173
foodways. *See* rural foodways and
localities; urban foodways
foodwork: aesthetics-driven, 148-51;
budget-driven, 143-47; in transnational and migrant families,
100, 186-88, 195, 199, 201; in vegetarian families, 103, 106, 109-11,
112-13, 114; of women and girls, 18,
64, 112, 199, 208, 229, 230
Foucault, Michel: discourse, 11, 13,
36-37, 38, 242; governmentality,
37, 54; technologies of the self, 38,
47, 121
France, 198-99
Fraser Valley (BC), 175, 178, 181. *See
also* British Columbia
frugality: healthy eating in conflict
with, 136-37; as necessity, 93, 143-
47; virtue and symbolic capital of,
155-56, 232, 233, 245

gardens: connection to food, 6, 173,
176, 178, 205-7; ethical eating and,
61, 71
gender: cosmopolitan eating repertoire and, 87; embodied tastes,
208-9; foodwork and, 18, 112;
going "underground," 231, 243;
healthy eating discourses and,
48-51, 230; logic of food practices
and, 229-31; macro-level body image discourse and, 132-33; men's
weight control, 129-33; in performance of ethnocultural identity, 188,
199, 200-201; and senses, 208;
vegetarianism and, 102-3; women's
weight control, 57, 123-29, 239. *See
also* fathers; femininity; masculine
foods; masculinity; men; mothers;
women
Giddens, Anthony, 11
global foods: appeal of Canadianized
versions of, 96-97; as healthy, 119;
in performance of ethnocultural

201, 237, 239; vegetarian eating
foodwork, 103, 106, 109-11, 112-13,
114
movement-space: about, 191; food
preparation and consumption as,
198-206; taste of home as, 192-98
multicultural neighbourhoods, 80,
89, 90-91, 171, 234

Nigerian foods, 193
Norman, Moss, 122-23
North American foods: appeal and
familiarity of, 96-97, 106-7; global-
ity and mobility of, 197, 202-3; meat-
and-potatoes as, 80, 83; in settlement workshops, 203; tentative
cosmopolitanism and, 96
North Riverdale (Toronto), 20(t), 64,
71
Northern foods, 168
Nova Scotia: about, 19, 20(t), 21;
global foods in, 81, 172, 181-82;
perceptions of rural foodways,
175-76, 176-77, 179, 182, 184-85;
traditional healthy eating discourse in, 44. *See also* Annapolis
Valley (NS); Halifax; Kings
County (NS)

obesity and fat: feminine framing of,
120-23, 221, 230; masculine framing of, 129-33, 221-22, 231; panic
surrounding, 7-8, 122, 133-34, 242;
rural areas associated with, 169,
183; techniques to discipline, 121-
23, 124-26; Western food as cause
of, 118
omnivorous eating, 83-84, 151, 237
Ontario: about, 20(t), 21; regional
cuisine, 168; rural foodways, 177-
79, 183. *See also* Kingston (ON);
Prince Edward County (ON);
Toronto
organic foods: cost of, 61, 73, 157, 173-
74, 215; in ethical eating repertoire,
61-62, 65-67, 71, 214; in healthy

eating discourse, 33-35, 41, 42, 59;
in Prince Edward County (ON),
163; on the superior taste of, 214,
215
Othering: bell hooks on, 84; cosmopolitan eating and, 216-17; Edward
Said on, 153; healthy eating discourse as form of, 152-55, 183, 233,
238, 243, 244, 246; Uma Narayan
on, 84; rural foodways and localities, 235, 236, 244; in settlement
cooking classes, 203-4

Pakistani cuisine and eating: gendered eating spaces and rhythms,
188, 200-1; taste of migration and
home, 186-87, 194, 197, 216
parents: conflict over children's body
image, 117, 223-25; enforcing
healthy eating, 54; parenting
vegetarian teens, 101, 105, 107-12;
transmit tastes and habitus, 209-
14, 220-21, 238
Pizza Hut, 194
place-based foodways: boundary
making through food, 28, 29; case
studies, 161-65; depicting rural
foodways, 168-69, 175-83, 184; depicting urban foodways, 168-69,
170-75, 184; eating repertoires
and, 9, 10, 44, 48, 80, 234; food
culture scenes, 71-72; mobile and
transnational, 189-90; regional
foodways in Canada, 167-68
pleasure: as danger, 221-22; food as,
138, 139, 147-51; as grounds to resist healthy eating, 34-35, 47-48,
225, 226
poverty and low income: alternative
ethical eating repertoire and, 74;
budget-driven food choices, 138,
139, 144-46, 147, 154; foods associated with, 136, 139, 152, 157; impact on healthy eating, 29, 60-61,
245; resistance to cosmopolitan
eating, 95-96

234; healthy eating in, 44. *See also*
British Columbia

vegetables: belonging and identity
and, 195-96, 198; as feminine, 48,
49, 51; as healthy, 33-34; poverty
associated with, 157

vegetarian eating: about, 102-3; case
studies, 99-101; class and, 102, 103,
104, 105-7, 109, 115, 232-33; culinary repertoires of, 105-7, 108, 115;
as embodied taste, 213; as ethical
eating, 28, 67-68, 73-74; foodwork
of, 103, 106, 109-10, 112-14; gendered, 102-3, 104; "good" parenting, 107-12; religion and, 74, 100,
109-10, 187; in sample, 103-4; teen
agency and, 110-14, 239

war on fat, 122, 242
Warde, Alan, 18
weight of foods, 49, 208-9
Weight Watchers, 124-25
whiteness, 26, 84, 236-37
women and girls: anti-obesity discourse critiqued by, 126-29, 242;
body image, 119-20, 123-29, 239;
the feminized body, 121-23, 208,
221; foodwork, 18, 64, 112, 199,
208, 229, 230; healthy eating and,
48-51, 230; husband's tastes, 188,
193-94; surveillance of food, 46-47,
128-29, 136, 156, 221; vegetarianism as feminine, 102-3. *See also*
mothers

ABOUT THE AUTHORS

Brenda Beagan
is a medical sociologist and associate professor in the
School of Occupational Therapy, Faculty of Health Professions,
Dalhousie University.

Gwen Chapman
is a professor in Food, Nutrition and Health in the Faculty of Land
and Food Systems, University of British Columbia.

Josée Johnston
is an associate professor in Sociology at the University of Toronto.

Deborah McPhail
is an assistant professor in Community Health Sciences in the
Faculty of Medicine, University of Manitoba.

Elaine M. Power
is an associate professor in the School of Kinesiology and
Health Studies at Queen's University, Kingston.

Helen Vallianatos
is an associate professor in the Department of Anthropology
at the University of Alberta.

Printed and bound in Canada by Friesens

Set in Eames, Sero, and Baskerville by Artegraphica Design Co. Ltd.

Copy editor: Deborah Kerr

Proofreader: Francis Chow

Indexer: Stephanie Watt